Jefferson
Headache Manual

Jefferson Headache Manual

William B. Young, MD, FAHS, FAAN
Associate Professor of Neurology
Director, Inpatient Program

Stephen D. Silberstein, MD, FACP
Professor of Neurology
Director, Jefferson Headache Center

Stephanie J. Nahas, MD
Assistant Professor of Neurology

Michael J. Marmura, MD
Assistant Professor of Neurology

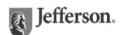 **Jefferson.**

Department of Neurology
Jefferson Headache Center
Thomas Jefferson University
Philadelphia, Pennsylvania

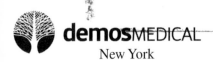
 demosMEDICAL
New York

Acquisitions Editor: Beth Barry
Cover Design: Joe Tenerelli
Compositor: NewGen
Printer: Hamilton Printing Company

Jefferson® is a registered trademark of Thomas Jefferson University. All rights reserved.

Visit our website at www.demosmedpub.com

Medicine is an ever-changing science. Research and clinical experience are continually expanding our knowledge, in particular our understanding of proper treatment and drug therapy. The authors, editors, and publisher have made every effort to ensure that all information in this book is in accordance with the state of knowledge at the time of production of the book. Nevertheless, the authors, editors, and publisher are not responsible for errors or omissions or for any consequences from application of the information in this book and make no warranty, express or implied, with respect to the contents of the publication. Every reader should examine carefully the package inserts accompanying each drug and should carefully check whether the dosage schedules mentioned therein or the contraindications stated by the manufacturer differ from the statements made in this book. Such examination is particularly important with drugs that are either rarely used or have been newly released on the market.

Library of Congress Cataloging-in-Publication Data

Jefferson headache manual / William B. Young ... [et al.].
    p. ; cm.
Headache manual
Includes bibliographical references and index.
ISBN 978-1-933864-70-9
    1. Headache—Diagnosis. 2. Headache—Treatment. I. Young, William B. (William Boyd), 1959–   II. Jefferson Headache Center.   III. Title: Headache manual. [DNLM:
1. Headache Disorders—diagnosis.   2. Headache Disorders—complications.
3. Headache Disorders—therapy. WL 342]
RC392.J44 2011
616.8'491—dc22   2010035585

Special discounts on bulk quantities of Demos Medical Publishing books are available to corporations, professional associations, pharmaceutical companies, health care organizations, and other qualifying groups. For details, please contact:
Special Sales Department
Demos Medical Publishing
11 W. 42nd Street, 15th Floor
New York, NY 10036
Phone: 800-532-8663 or 212-683-0072
Fax: 212-941-7842
E-mail: rsantana@demosmedpub.com

Made in the United States of America
10 11 12   13   14   5 4 3 2 1

Contents

Preface

The prevalence, societal costs, and intricacies of headache disorders are extremely high. Despite this, research that would help in the care and management of headache patients is sadly lacking. Almost every patient who seeks treatment at our headache center has failed most Food and Drug Administration-approved treatments, or there *are* no Food and Drug Administration-approved treatments for his or her said disorder. Headache patients often do not get a diagnosis, do not achieve effective acute pain relief, and do not receive preventive therapy. The National Institutes of Health have provided limited resources for basic headache research. Few clinical trials have been done, despite the fact that headache afflicts millions of Americans.

When the patient's symptoms are dire, we refuse to abandon the patient to treatment nihilism and endless pain, and are forced to go beyond the meager offerings of evidence-based medicine. We have come up with our own empirical techniques. We talk among ourselves and to other headache experts. We meet, dissect our results, review our adverse events, try to improve our patients' lives, and attempt to get funding to prove our beliefs.

This manual is a practical guide that aims to give the reader a sense of how headache medicine is actually practiced and why we do what we do. If one were writing a manual on cardiac care, one would have standards to quote, erudite discussions in the literature on even rarely used aggressive treatments, and consensus conferences to cite on various issues. An excellent manual, both practical and scientific, could arise based upon this literature. But for headache medicine, a scant volume would emerge, useless for the patients who populate our clinics.

We hope this manual will assist you in the care of your patients. We hope you will keep this book close at hand, and let it serve as a quick reference when new treatments are contemplated, or when you know what to do but not how to do it. In the future, new treatments will emerge and be studied scientifically. But for now, we believe this book is pretty close to the "state of the art" of headache medicine.

William B. Young, MD, FAHS, FAAN
Stephen D. Silberstein, MD, FACP
Stephanie J. Nahas, MD
Michael J. Marmura, MD

Acknowledgments

Our thanks and appreciation to Linda Kelly for her excellent organizational skills, to Lynne Kaiser for her editorial proficiency, and to both of them for their dedication and commitment.

Jefferson
Headache Manual

1 Classification of Headache: How and Why—Primary versus Secondary Headache

Classification helps us better diagnose headache disorders and ultimately treat them properly. The International Headache Society classification has three parts—primary headaches, secondary headaches, and cranial neuralgias (Table 1.1). Primary headaches are those in which the headache itself is the disorder. Secondary headaches are caused by structural, inflammatory, or metabolic problems. Cranial neuralgias are head pains caused or behaving as if they were due to stimulation, compression, or distortion of a nerve of the head.

Migraine is the most important primary headache (Table 1.2). It is subclassified into migraine with and without aura. Most people who have migraine do not have aura, but about 30% do.

Migraine is diagnosed clinically. There is no test and no practical way to prove that a headache is a migraine, other than by eliciting its symptoms and excluding a secondary cause. Sometimes patients forget to read the rule book. For example, they may be missing just one of the features. First this was called "migrainous headache." Later it was renamed "probable migraine." These semantics serve little function, because for all practical purposes, "probable migraine" responds to the same treatment as ICHD-II migraine.

The pathophysiology of migraine aura is becoming better understood, but there is no practical test other than the clinical features to diagnose aura. This is problematic because other neurologic conditions can cause similar symptoms. If a person has migraine with typical visual aura, no evaluation is necessary. These are so characteristic and common that in the absence of

TABLE 1.1 Examples of Primary and Secondary Headaches

Primary Headaches	Secondary Headaches	Cranial Neuralgias
Migraine	Brain tumor headache	Trigeminal neuralgia
Tension-type headache	Cervicogenic headache	Glossopharyngeal neuralgia
Cluster headache	Headache associated with fever	Persistent idiopathic facial pain

TABLE 1.2 ICHD-II Criteria for Migraine

A. At least five attacks fulfilling criteria B-D
B. Headache attacks lasting 4 to 72 hours (untreated or unsuccessfully treated)
C. Headache has ≥2 of the following characteristics:
　　1. Unilateral location
　　2. Pulsating quality
　　3. Moderate or severe pain intensity
　　4. Aggravation by or causing avoidance of routine physical activity
　　　(e.g., walking, climbing stairs)
D. During headache ≥1 of the following can occur:
　　1. Nausea and/or vomiting
　　2. Photophobia and phonophobia
E. Not attributed to another disorder

red flags, no further studies are needed beyond the history and examination. If the aura is atypical (involving severe language dysfunction, weakness, or other unusual symptoms), brain and blood vessel imaging may be necessary (Table 1.3).

Be aware of aggravating factors. Often a patient will have a primary headache worsened by something else. Sometimes this is a bad habit or modifiable lifestyle issue: sleep better, kick your mother-in-law out of the house. Other times it is a medical condition requiring a hypothesis, testing, and treatment: get the sleep apnea test, find the cervical facet disease or temporomandibular joint dysfunction, and see the psychiatrist for your major depression—treat these disorders and the migraine will often improve.

The final part of the classification is the cranial neuralgias. They are less common and are separated out for a few reasons: (1) pain predominates far more than other neurologic symptoms, (2) etiology often can be attributed fairly directly to damage or irritation of a peripheral nerve, and (3) treatments for these disorders often differ from those for other primary headaches.

TABLE 1.3 Diagnostic Criteria for Migraine Aura

- At least two attacks
- Aura consisting of ≥1 of the following, but no motor weakness:
　　1. Fully reversible visual symptoms including positive and/or negative features
　　2. Fully reversible sensory symptoms including positive and/or negative features
　　3. Fully reversible dysphasic speech disturbance

In this book, we hope to cover a wide range of diagnoses and treatments, not necessarily exhaustively, but deeply enough, to make you comfortable in practicing safely.

REFERENCE

Headache Classification Committee. The International Classification of Headache Disorders: 2nd edition. *Cephalalgia.* 2004;24(suppl 1):9–160.

2 Headache Epidemiology

Migraine occurs throughout the human life span. The youngest age of migraine onset is hard to determine. We have had many parents tell us of their very young, nonverbal child who becomes pale and fussy; then cries, vomits, sleeps, and returns to normal. When the child gets older and learns to speak, he or she verbalizes that these spells are accompanied by severe headache.

Migraine occurs at an overall rate of 12% (18% of females and 6% of males). "Probable migraine," also known as migrainous headache, has an overall 1-year prevalence of 4.5%. Migraine may be more common in young boys than young girls. Once menarche begins, girls develop migraine at a ratio that approximates 3.5 to 1. The prevalence of migraine through the life span is illustrated in Figures 2.1 and 2.2.

Overall, migraine prevalence has been stable from 1997 to 2007. Household income is inversely proportional to the prevalence of migraine, with persons in the lowest bracket having 1.6 times the rate of migraine as persons in the highest socioeconomic bracket. After adjustments for income, whites have more migraines than blacks, who, in turn, have more than Asians.

Chronic migraine is present in 2% to 3% of the US population. In population-based studies, people appear to evolve to chronic migraine at a rate of about 3% and out of chronic migraine also at a rate of about 3% per year.

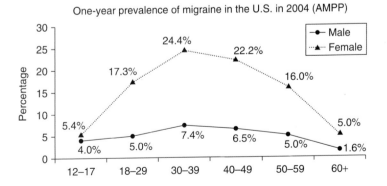

FIGURE 2.1 Migraine prevalence by age.

Source: Lipton RB, et al. *Neurology*. 2007;68:343–349.

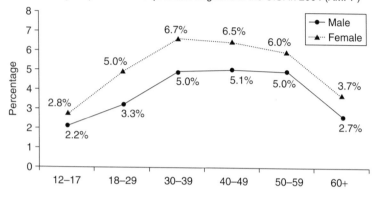

FIGURE 2.2 Probable migraine prevalence by age.
Source: Silberstein S, et al. *Cephalalgia*. 2007;27:220–229.

Migraine ranks as the 20th most disabling (on a population basis) condition in industrialized countries.

Episodic tension-type headache is present in about 46% of the US population, and chronic tension-type headache is present in approximately 2%. However, individuals with tension-type headaches do not show up very often in the doctor's office. In primary care offices, a person who complains of recurring headache has a 94% chance of having migraine or probable migraine, and most of the rest have tension-type headache.

Cluster headache occurs in 53 persons per 100,000 in the population. The male-female ratio is 4.3, although this gap may be narrowing. Six times as many people have episodic cluster headache as have chronic cluster. In the tertiary care setting, many patients self-identify as being "epichronic," whereby, under the influence of continuous treatment, they have periods of incomplete control with infrequent or less intense attacks without prolonged periods of remission. Age of onset varies in the literature from 3 to 91 years, with the reported mean age of onset between 26 and 30 years.

RESEARCH AND INVESTMENT

The burden of headache disorders is enormous and their treatment is not well-financed or understood. Migraine headaches alone result in more than 1% of the total disability burden in the United States. The US government spends less money per hours of migraine-related disability than for almost any medical disease (Figure 2.3).

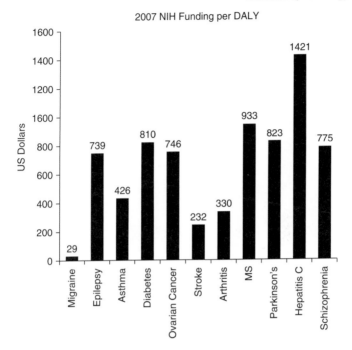

FIGURE 2.3 Amount of research of money spent by National Institutes of Health (NIH) per disability-adjusted life year (DALY).

REFERENCES

Fischera M, Marziniak M, Gralow I, Evers S. The incidence and prevalence of cluster headache: a meta-analysis of population-based studies. *Cephalalgia.* 2008;28(6):614–618.

Lipton RB, Bigal M, Diamond M. Migraine prevalence, disease burden and the need for preventive therapy. *Neurology.* 2007;68:343–349.

Schwedt TJ, Shapiro RE. Funding of research on headache disorders by the National Institutes of Health. *Headache.* 2009;49(2):162–169.

Silberstein S, Loder E, Diamond S, et al; AMPP Advisory Group. Probable migraine in the United States: results of the American Migraine Prevalence and Prevention (AMPP) study. *Cephalalgia.* 2007;27:220–234.

Tepper SJ, Dahlof CG, Dowson A, et al. Prevalence and diagnosis of migraine in patients consulting their physician with a complaint of headache: data from the landmark study. *Headache.* 2004;44(9):856–864.

3 Diagnosis and Testing of Primary and Secondary Headache

THE HEADACHE HISTORY AND EXAMINATION

The headache physician relies less on diagnostic testing than on the history, and physical examination. The headache history requires exploring specific areas and the physical examination requires developing new skills. A headache patient's history should explore the temporal course of the illness and the presence of symptoms that the patient may not think are important: "Why should I mention my mild daily headaches that I suppress with aspirin? They don't bother me."

One needs to ask what effect the headache has on the patient's life and what disability it has caused. Ask an open-ended question, such as "How do your headaches affect your life?" early in the interview. Give the patient time to consider the question and answer it before moving on. This improves patient satisfaction and actually shortens the interaction.

We concentrate on the following items on initial evaluation of the headache patient.

- Headache onset
  - Age at onset
  - Factors associated with onset
    - Namely, Valsalva, sex, exercise, a febrile illness
- Location of pain
  - Nonspecific: primary and secondary headaches can be unilateral or bilateral
  - Occipital headache could be ominous in a child, but usually not in an adult
- Duration of pain: migraine 4+ hours, cluster <3 hours
- Frequency and timing of attacks
  - Cluster–multiple daily attacks
- Pain severity and course
  - Was onset sudden?
  - Was course progressive, relentless?
- Quality of pain
  - Throbbing, stabbing, burning, and so on.
    - Least important factor

- Aggravating/relieving factors
  - Body position (orthostatic)
  - Head movement
- Associated features
  - Migraine (nausea, photo- and phonophobia)
  - Cluster headache (eye-tearing, restlessness)
- Medical history
  - Medications
  - Disorders affecting teeth, sinuses, or surrounding tissues
  - Prior lumbar puncture
  - Head trauma
  - Carcinoma
  - Epilepsy
  - HIV
- Physical examination (body as a whole)
  - Vital signs
  - Head—examine scars, areas of previous trauma for tenderness, or Tinel's sign
  - Temporomandibular joints—palpate the joint, feel for clicks and lateral movements during opening, assure that patient can open wide enough for three (of his or her own) fingers
  - Neck and shoulders—trigger points, range of motion, stress the facets and discs by hyperextending the laterally tipped head
  - Muscles and tendons
  - Skin
- Neurologic examination (usually normal in primary headache disorder)
  - Funduscopic examination
  - Mental status
  - Cranial nerves
  - Motor system
  - Reflexes
  - Coordination
  - Gait
  - Sensory system

Some patients with a complaint of headache may require additional investigations. The SNOOP mnemonic, developed by the American Headache Society, is taught to residents and medical students throughout the country (Table 3.1). The presence of any of these signs or symptoms is a red flag and indicates the need to perform a more extensive evaluation.

Headache evaluation begins with a search for red flags (Figure 3.1). This is the medicolegal minimum for evaluating a patient for the first time or evaluating a patient with a new or changed headache.

TABLE 3.1 Worrisome Headache Red Flags ("SNOOP")

- **S**ystemic symptoms (fever, weight loss) or **S**econdary risk factors (HIV, systemic cancer)
- **N**eurologic symptoms or abnormal signs (impaired alertness or consciousness, confusion)
- **O**nset: sudden, abrupt, or split-second
- **O**lder: new-onset and progressive headache, especially in middle age (> 50 [giant cell arteritis])
- **P**revious headache history: different headache (marked change in attack frequency, severity, or clinical features)

See Chapter 12 for more details.

DIAGNOSIS AND TESTING

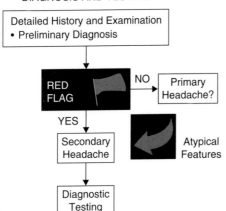

FIGURE 3.1 When to test.

IMAGING IN HEADACHE EVALUATION

Computerized tomography (CT) will detect many abnormalities that can cause headaches. It is equal or superior to magnetic resonance imaging (MRI) to diagnose acute subarachnoid hemorrhage (SAH), acute head trauma, and bony abnormalities. Head CT may miss many vascular, neoplastic, cervicomedullary, and infectious disorders (Table 3.2).

MRI in Migraine

Migraineurs have more posterior infarct-like lesion than nonmigraineurs (5.4% vs 0.7%). The risk varies by migraine subtype and attack frequency. The highest risk is in migraineurs with aura experiencing one attack or more per month. Focal (possibly migraine-related) hypoperfusion rather than

TABLE 3.2 Causes of Headache That Can be Missed on Routine CT Scan of the Head

Vascular disease	■ Meningeal carcinomatosis
■ Aneurysm	■ Pituitary tumor or hemorrhage
■ AVM (especially posterior fossa)	***Cervicomedullary lesions***
■ SAH	■ Chiari malformation
■ Carotid or vertebral artery dissection	■ Foramen magnum meningioma
■ Infarct (especially early)	***Infections***
■ Cerebral venous thrombosis	■ Paranasal sinusitis
■ Vasculitis	■ Meningoencephalitis
■ White matter abnormalities	■ Cerebritis and brain abscess
■ Subdural and epidural hematoma	***Other***
Neoplastic disease	■ Low CSF pressure/volume syndrome
■ Neoplasm (especially in posterior fossa)	■ Idiopathic hypertrophic pachymeningitis

Abbreviations: AVM, arteriovenous malformation; CSF, cerebrospinal fluid; CT, computerized tomography; SAH, subarachnoid hemorrhage.
Source: Evans RW. Headaches. In: *Diagnostic Testing in Neurology*. Philadelphia, PA: W. B. Saunders; 1999:3.

microembolic occlusion may be responsible for most cerebellar lesions (Figure 3.2).

Thirty-eight percent of subjects with or without migraine had at least one medium-sized deep white matter lesion (DWML) (Figure 3.3). Among

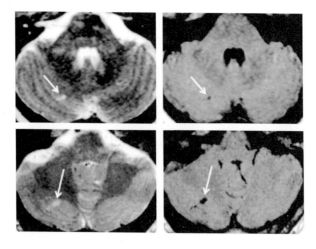

FIGURE 3.2 Cerebellar infarct.

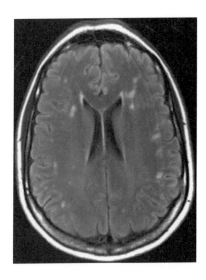

FIGURE 3.3 Subcortical white matter abnormalities.

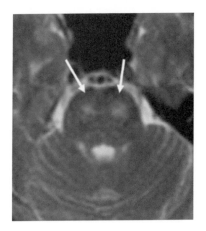

FIGURE 3.4 Pontine hyperintense lesions.

women, the risk for high DWML load was increased in migraineurs; this risk increased with attack frequency, being highest in those with at least one attack per month (OR, 2.6) but similar in patients with migraine with or without aura. In men, controls and patients with migraine did not differ in DWML prevalence. Kruit et al. also found brainstem and dorsal basis pontis hyperintense lesions in their migraine population. They were identified in 13 of 295 migraineurs (4.4%) and in 1 of 140 controls (0.7%) (Figure 3.4).

Migraine-like headaches with atypical visual symptoms can rarely be associated with occipital lobe arteriovenous malformations (AVMs).

MRI in Cluster Headache

Patients with cluster headaches usually have normal MRIs. However, atypical cluster headache may have a secondary cause. Some authorities believe that a secondary cause of cluster headache may rarely be found even in typical cluster headache cases (Table 3.3).

TABLE 3.3 Differential Diagnoses of Cluster Headache

Primary Headache Syndromes
- Paroxysmal hemicrania
- SUNCT
- Hemicrania continua
- Migraine
- Hypnic headache

Secondary Causes of Cluster Headache
Vascular causes
- Carotid or vertebral artery dissection or aneurysm
- Pseudoaneurysm of intracavernous carotid artery
- Anterior communicating artery aneurysm
- Occipital lobe AVM
- Middle cerebral artery territory AVM
- AVM in soft tissue of scalp above ear
- Frontal lobe and corpus callosum AVM
- Cervical cord infarction
- Lateral medullary infarction
- Frontotemporal subdural hematoma

Tumors
- Pituitary tumors
- Parasellar meningioma
- Sphenoidal meningioma
- Epidermoid tumor in the prepontine (behind the dorsum sella turcica)
- Tentorial meningioma
- High cervical meningioma
- Nasopharyngeal carcinoma

Infectious causes
- Maxillary sinusitis
- Orbitosphenoidal aspergillosis
- Herpes zoster ophthalmicus

Posttrauma or postsurgery
- Facial trauma
- Following enucleation of eye

Dental causes
- Infected wisdom tooth
- Dental extraction

Miscellaneous
- Cervical syringomyelia and Chiari malformation
- IIH

Secondary headache syndromes
- Tolosa-Hunt syndrome
- Temporal arteritis
- Raeder's paratrigeminal neuralgia

Abbreviations: AVM, arteriovenous malformation; IIH, idiopathic intracranial hypertension; SUNCT, short-lasting unilateral neuralgiform headache attacks with conjunctival injection and tearing.

Source: Matharu and Goadsby. *Wolff's Headache and Other Head Pain*. 8th ed. New York, NY: Oxford University Press; 2008.

Radiation Exposure and the Pregnant Patient

A dose of 15 rads may result in deformities that might justify pregnancy termination. With lead shielding, a standard CT scan of the head exposes the uterus to less than 1 mrad. The radiation dose for a typical cervical or intracranial arteriogram is less than 1 mrad. MRI during pregnancy has no known risk, but its use during pregnancy is controversial because the magnets raise the body's core temperature (less than 1°C). Pregnant MRI workers were not found to have adverse fetal outcomes, and no adverse fetal effects from MRI have been documented to date. MRI, like all imaging techniques, should be used only when the benefits outweigh the risks. Contrast should be avoided if possible. The American College of Obstetricians and Gynecologists' guidelines on the use of diagnostic imaging modalities during pregnancy state that MRI is not associated with known adverse fetal defects; they recommend avoiding contrast agents, however, unless medically necessary for the mother.

Electroencephalography

The only significant abnormality reported in studies with a relatively acceptable design was prominent driving in response to photic stimulation (the "H-response") in migraineurs. This finding is not necessary for the clinical diagnosis of migraine. The report of the Quality Standards Subcommittee of the American Academy of Neurology suggests the following practice parameter: "The electroencephalogram (EEG) is not useful in the routine evaluation of patients with headache. This does not exclude the use of EEG to evaluate headache patients with associated symptoms suggesting a seizure disorder, such as atypical migrainous aura or episodic loss of consciousness."

Lumbar Puncture

MRI or CT scan is usually performed before an LP, except in cases where acute bacterial meningitis is suspected. LP can be diagnostic for SAH, meningitis or encephalitis, meningeal carcinomatosis or lymphomatosis, and low or high (e.g., idiopathic intracranial hypertension [IIH]) cerebrospinal fluid (CSF) pressure (Table 3.4). LP is indicated when any of the following are present: the sudden onset of the worst headache of a patient's life; headache with fever or other symptoms or signs suggesting an infectious cause; a HIV-positive patient or a person with carcinoma with a subacute or progressive headache; an atypical chronic headache (e.g., to rule out IIH in an obese woman even without papilledema); and a headache that has not responded to typical medication regimes.

TABLE 3.4 Approximate Probability of Recognizing SAH on CT Scan after the Initial Event

Time	Probability (%)
Day 0	95
Day 3	74
1 week	50
2 weeks	30
3 weeks	Almost 0

Abbreviations: CT, computerized tomography; SAH, subarachnoid hemorrhage.

Source: Evans RW. Headaches. In: *Diagnostic Testing in Neurology*. Philadelphia, PA: W. B. Saunders; 1999:9.

CSF EXAMINATION AND XANTHOCHROMIA

Red blood cells (RBCs) are seen in the CSF in virtually all cases of SAH and clear in about 6 to 30 days. Distinguishing a traumatic LP from an SAH can be problematic. Although the RBC count is usually high and is stable or rises in sequential tubes, fewer than 100 RBCs may still indicate SAH, and a 25% reduction between the first and last tubes can be seen in SAH. Crenated RBCs are not a reliable sign of SAH (Table 3.5).

TABLE 3.5 Causes of Nontraumatic SAH

Intracranial aneurysm (most common)
Intracranial AVM
Benign perimesencephalic hemorrhage
Other causes:
■ Vertebral or carotid artery dissection
■ Dural AVM
■ Spinal AVM
■ Sickle cell anemia
■ Coagulation disorders
■ Drug abuse (cocaine and methamphetamine)
■ Primary or metastatic intracranial tumors (e.g., pituitary, melanoma)
■ Primary or metastatic cervical tumors
■ CNS infection (e.g., herpes encephalitis)
■ CNS vasculitides

Abbreviations: AVM, arteriovenous malformation; CNS, central nervous system; SAH, subarachnoid hemorrhage.

Source: Evans RW. Headaches. In: *Diagnostic Testing in Neurology*. Philadelphia, PA: W. B. Saunders; 1999:7.

When RBCs break down in the CSF, they release oxyhemoglobin, which is degraded to bilirubin by 3 to 4 days. These two agents are responsible for CSF xanthochromia. The CSF supernatant is pink or pink-orange due to oxyhemoglobin, yellow due to bilirubin, and an intermediate color if both are present. Although oxyhemoglobin can be detected as early as 2 hours after entry of RBCs into CSF, xanthochromia is often not present for 12 hours. Some authorities suggest delaying LP until 12 hours after the ictus. This is not always practical and can delay the diagnosis. The presence of xanthochromia on spectrophotometry cannot always distinguish between SAH and a traumatic LP (Table 3.6).

Because oxyhemoglobin can form in vivo, false-positives for SAH can occur from traumatic taps. Assess CSF xanthochromia by spectrophotometry within 2 hours after traumatic LP and sooner in samples with more than 10,000 RBCs/ mm3. In contrast, xanthochromia in traumatic LP with fewer than 5000 RBCs warrants further investigation for SAH. The naked eye can only detect xanthochromia about half the time. The clinical utility of spectrophotometry is debatable because of false positives. Fewer than 1% of patients with oxyhemoglobin alone had aneurysms diagnosed, whereas 21% of patients with bilirubin had an aneurysm (Table 3.7).

TABLE 3.6 The Probability of Detecting Xanthochromia with Spectrophotometry in the CSF at Various Times after an SAH

Time	Probability (%)
12 hours	100
1 week	100
2 weeks	100
3 weeks	More than 70
4 weeks	More than 40

Abbreviations: CSF, cerebrospinal fluid; SAH, subarachnoid hemorrhage.
Source: Vermeulen M, et al. *J Neurol Neurosurg Psychiatr*. 1989;52:826–828.

TABLE 3.7 Other Causes of Xanthochromia

- Jaundice (usually with a total plasma bilirubin of 10 to 15 mg/dl)
- CSF protein more than 150 mg/dl
- Dietary hypercarotenemia
- Malignant melanomatosis
- Oral intake of rifampin
- Traumatic LP

Abbreviations: CSF, cerebrospinal fluid; LP, lumbar puncture.

WHAT ELSE MIGHT BE GOING ON

Acute medication overuse is often missed (Chapter 9). Retake the medication history, asking about over-the-counter medications that the patient may have neglected to mention; you may need to question the spouse or family members, check urine toxicology screens, and consider whether a patient may be multi-sourcing prescription medications. Secondary headaches that are commonly missed are listed in Table 3.8.

IIH with papilledema (pseudotumor cerebri) may occur, and it is critical to examine the optic discs of all patients with a new headache. IIH without papilledema can be a difficult diagnosis because there are no distinguishing headache features, although patients may have pulsatile tinnitus or an abducens nerve palsy. They do not get true visual obscurations, but may still have vague visual complaints. IIH with or without papilledema usually occurs in adult women with a body mass index (BMI) more than 30. Clues on MRI include an empty sella. The magnetic resonance venography (MRV) may show lateral sinus stenosis. If IIH is diagnosed, look for medications that can cause this syndrome, such as minocycline.

A number of exogenous substances may cause headache (Table 3.9). Special mention should be made of carbon monoxide poisoning, which usually presents with mild headaches without gastrointestinal or neurologic symptoms, unless carboxyhemoglobin levels are high.

Low CSF pressure headache may be caused by a cryptogenic, rhinogenic, or spinal leak, the latter being more common. An orthostatic headache is usually present, but low CSF pressure headache has other presentations (Table 3.10). Early on, the headache is postural, but the postural characteristics may be lost.

Characteristic MRI findings include diffuse pachymeningeal enhancement (with gadolinium), sagging of the hindbrain (including secondary [reversible] Chiari), subdural collections (including spinal and cerebral hygromas and

TABLE 3.8 Undiagnosed Secondary Headache

■ Medication overuse	■ Chronic meningitis
■ Giant cell arteritis	■ Metabolic disorders
■ Carotid dissection	■ Mediastinal process
■ IIH/pseudotumor	• Angina
■ Low pressure headache	• Mass lesions
■ Chronic sphenoid sinusitis	• Superior vena cava syndrome
■ Nasopharyngeal carcinoma	■ Primary trochlear headache and trochleitis
■ Subacute angle closure glaucoma	■ Cervicogenic headache—facet disease

Abbreviation: IIH, idiopathic intracranial hypertension.

TABLE 3.9 Medications That Could Induce Headache

Acyclovir	Histamine blockers
Adalimumab	■ Cimetidine
Albendazole	■ Ranitidine
Alpha methyldopa	Interferon (1a and 1b)
Amphotericin	■ Alpha 2a
Atovaquone	■ Alpha 2b
Bromocriptine	■ Beta 1a
Chloroquine	■ Beta 1b
Cyclosporine	Nitric oxide donors
Desmopressin	■ Amyl nitrate
Disulfiram	■ Isosorbide mono- or dinitrate
Etanercept	■ Nitroglycerin
Griseofulvin	■ Sodium nitroprusside
Hydralazine	Oxytocin
Hydroxychloroquine	Phosphodiesterase inhibitors
Indomethacin	■ Dipyridamole
Infliximab	■ Sildenafil
Isotretinoin	Quinalones
Linezolid	■ Ciprofloxacin
Lithium	■ Norfloxacin
Lopinavir	■ Ofloxacin, etc.
Muromonab/CD3	Serotonin antagonists
Naltrexone	■ Granisetron
Nifedipine	■ Odansetron
Nimodipine	
Nonsteroidal antiinflammatory drugs	
Phenylpropanolomine	
Praziquantel	
Progestins	
Ritonavir	
Sulfasalazine	
Tetracycline	
Vitamin A	
Zidovuzone	

hematomas), pituitary enlargement, and enlarged spinal and cerebral veins. The LP usually shows low CSF pressure. Pleocytosis or increased protein may be present (Chapter 16).

Certain headache characteristics are worrisome and require a specific workup. These include thunderclap headache, rapidly progressive headache, new daily persistent headache (NDPH), and postural or orthostatic headache. Focal pain and headache may evoke a specific differential diagnosis and a

TABLE 3.10 Spontaneous Low CSF Pressure Headache

- Rhinogenic vs spinal leak
- Orthostatic headache
- Characteristic MRI findings
  - Diffuse pachymeningeal enhancement
  - Sagging hindbrain
  - Subdural collection
  - Pituitary enlargement
- LP findings
  - Low CSF pressure (less than 100 mm H_2O)
  - Possible pleocytosis
  - Possible increased protein

Abbreviations: CSF, cerebrospinal fluid; LP, lumbar puncture; MRI, magnetic resonance imaging.

TABLE 3.11 Migraine with Neurologic Symptoms

- Basilar migraine
- Vertiginous migraine
- Confusional migraine
- Ophthalmoplegic migraine[a]
- Hemiplegic migraine (familial or sporadic)
- MUMS (migraine with unilateral motor symptoms)
- CADASIL (cerebral autosomal dominant arteriopathy with subcortical infarcts and leukoencephalopathy)
- Alternating hemiplegia of childhood
- Ornithine transcarbamylase deficiency

[a] Now considered a cranial neuralgia.

specific diagnostic workup. These include headache associated with eye pain, pain or symptoms referable to the sinus or nose, severe neck pain, and pain in the teeth, mouth, or jaw.

Migraine can occur with unusual neurologic symptoms. In the presence of a normal interictal neurologic examination, it is usually a primary headache. Differential diagnoses are given in Table 3.11.

THUNDERCLAP HEADACHE

A thunderclap headache may be defined as a headache that reaches maximum severe intensity in less than 1 minute. This is conservative, as most thunderclap headaches are nearly instantaneous. The differential diagnosis for thunderclap headache is listed in Table 3.12. SAH is the most common secondary cause of a

TABLE 3.12 Differential Diagnosis for Thunderclap Headache

■ SAH	■ Acute hypertensive crisis
■ Sentinel headache	■ Reversible cerebral
■ Cerebral venous sinus thrombosis	vasoconstriction syndrome
■ Cervical artery dissection	■ Third ventricle colloid cyst
■ Spontaneous intracranial hypotension	■ Intracranial infection
■ Pituitary apoplexy	■ Primary thunderclap headache
■ Retroclival hematoma	■ Primary cough, sexual, and
■ Ischemic stroke	exertional headache

Abbreviation: SAH, subarachnoid hemorrhage.

thunderclap headache and should be evaluated as rapidly as possible. Patients seen in the first few hours should have a CT scan and, if the CT is negative, an LP. Other causes of thunderclap headache are listed in Table 3.12. Most can be diagnosed with MRI, *magnetic resonance angiography (*MRA), or MRV. In some cases, CT angiogram (CTA) may be needed.

Primary thunderclap headache is a diagnosis of exclusion. It is usually very severe, lasts less than 1 week, and then gradually fades away. Primary thunderclap headache may be clinically indistinguishable from a reversible cerebral vascular syndrome or Call-Fleming syndrome. Individuals who have a thunderclap headache with a normal CT and LP should have an MRA or CTA performed as soon as possible. A number of complications often occur late in the course of reversible cerebral vasoconstriction syndromes (Figure 3.5, Table 3.13). Some patients may not have vasospasm on the first MRA, but have vasospasm on a second MRA several days after thunderclap headache onset. One clue to reversible cerebral vasoconstriction syndromes is recurrent thunderclap headaches. We generally do not recommend a formal angiogram, as it may promote vasospasm.

PROGRESSIVE RAPIDLY WORSENING HEADACHE

A differential diagnosis of rapidly progressive headache is presented in Table 3.14. Any mass lesion, including extra-axial collections, such as epidural and subdural hematomas, abscesses, or empyemas, may cause this. Intra-axial mass lesions usually have more prominent neurologic findings. Occasionally, extracranial lesions, particularly apical lung disorders, present with head or facial pain. Sphenoid sinusitis may present with a thunderclap or rapidly progressive headache. Giant cell arteritis, venous sinus thrombosis, meningitis, and encephalitis can present with a headache that evolves rapidly; some (e.g., venous sinus thrombosis) may present with a thunderclap onset.

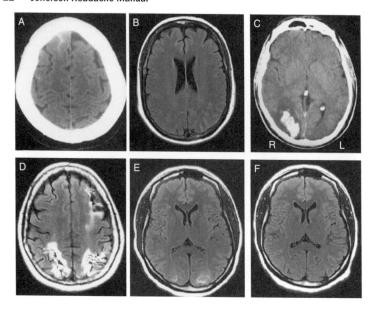

FIGURE 3.5 Brain imaging in reversible cerebral vasoconstriction syndromes (RCVS). (A) CT scan showing a small cortical SAH, (B) MRI (fluid-attenuated inversion recovery sequence) showing a small cortical SAH, (C) CT scan showing an occipital intracerebral hemorrhage, (D) MRI showing sequelae of bilateral occipital infarcts and left frontal-parietal infarct, (E) MRI (fluid-attenuated inversion recovery) showing hypersignals consistent with a reversible posterior leukoencephalopathy syndrome, and (F) control MRI in the same patient after 28 days showing resolution of the reversible posterior leukoencephalopathy syndrome.

TABLE 3.13 Mean Delay from Headache Onset to Other Features of Reversible Cerebral Vasoconstriction Syndromes

Delay from Headache Onset to Diagnosis	Number of Cases	Mean ± SD (days)	Range (days)
Intracerebral hemorrhage	4	1.7 ± 2	0–4
SAH	15	5 ± 5	0–20
First seizure	2	3 ± 1.4	2–4
Reversible posterior leukoencephalopathy syndrome	6	4 ± 1.9	1–6
Last recurrent thunderclap headache	63	7.4 ± 5.6	0–28
Transient neurologic deficit	11	11.6 ± 4.9	0–23
Diagnosis of cerebral infarction	3	12 ± 3	9–15

Abbreviation: SAH, subarachnoid hemorrhage.
Source: Ducros A, Boukobza M, Porcher R, et al. *Brain.* 2007;130:3091–3101.

TABLE 3.14 Rapidly Progressive Headache Differential

- Any mass lesion
  - Intra-axial
  - Extra-axial
  - Extracranial
- Sphenoid sinusitis
- Giant cell arteritis
- Venous sinus thrombosis
- Meningitis
- Encephalitis

NEW DAILY PERSISTENT HEADACHE

NDPH (Table 3.15) is a primary headache that occurs daily from onset. Triggering events, most commonly a flu-like or viral prodrome, are found in approximately one-third of patients. Occasionally, a specific viral etiology, such as Epstein-Barr virus, is identified. Lyme disease is treatable, and testing for this disorder should be considered (except when exposure is unlikely to have occurred). Venous sinus thrombosis, high and low CSF pressure syndromes, and chronic meningitis may present as NDPH. Our usual minimal evaluation of patients with NDPH and a normal neurologic examination is an MRI with gadolinium, an MRV, and a Lyme titer (if endemic). If an initial round of treatment is ineffective, an LP may be appropriate.

TABLE 3.15 NDPH Differential

- Venous sinus thrombosis
- IIH
- Low pressure headache (CSF leak)
- Carotid or vertebral artery dissection
- Meningitis (Lyme, fungal, TB, HIV)
- Sphenoid sinusitis
- Posttraumatic headache
- Cervical facet syndrome
- Intranasal contact point headache

Abbreviations: CSF, cerebrospinal fluid; IIH, idiopathic intracranial hypertension; NDPH, new daily persistent headache.

ORTHOSTATIC HEADACHE

Orthostatic headache is often due to low CSF pressure caused by a spinal CSF leak (e.g., LP or cryptogenic). Less commonly, it may be caused by a cranial CSF leak (e.g., CSF rhinorrhea). Occasionally, a mass with a ball-valve type of effect—most commonly a colloid cyst—may present as postural headache, although this headache is not generally orthostatic. A postural headache can occur with dysautonomia (POTS = postural orthostatic tachycardia syndrome), which is diagnosed with a tilt table test. In some cases, all testing is normal, and the etiology of orthostatic phenomena is unclear.

EYE PAIN AND HEADACHE

Headache may be located in or near the eye; this phenomenon has its own differential diagnosis and evaluation. Many eye disorders can cause pain; most are not neurologic diagnostic challenges. An ophthalmologic etiology is usually obvious, because the eye examination is typically abnormal. Headache with eye pain (with a normal eye examination) is most likely because of migraine but also occurs in other primary headache disorders, such as cluster headache, hemicrania continua, paroxysmal hemicrania, short-lasting unilateral neuralgiform headache attacks with conjunctival injection and tearing (SUNCT), short-lasting unilateral neuralgiform headache attacks with cranial autonomic features (SUNA), V1 trigeminal neuralgia, and idiopathic stabbing headache. Causes of headache with eye pain without obvious cranial nerve abnormalities are listed in Table 3.16.

Behçet and Vogt-Koyanagi Harada syndromes are common causes of uveitis with headache. Inflammatory processes or tumors of the orbit may also present with headache. Trochleitis and primary trochlear headache presenting with chronic daily headache, with pain referable to the eye or to the inner canthus

TABLE 3.16 Other Causes of Headache Associated with Eye Pain

- Angle closure glaucoma
  - Pain as pressure rises
  - Dilated or irregular pupil during attacks
  - May have migrainous features: nausea and vomiting
- Trochleitis
  - Inflammation of the trochlea, tenderness on examination
  - Painful supraduction
  - Idiopathic rheumatoid arthritis, systemic lupus erythematosis, psoriasis, and enteric arthropathy
  - Baseline pain in inner aspect of eye, exacerbates migraine
- Primary trochlear headache
  - Pain in trochlear area, other areas in 60%
  - Imaging normal
  - Local steroids successful in 95%, also help concurrent headache
  - Relapses in 45%, average 8 months
- Dry eye syndrome
- Uveitis

area, has been described. Cavernous sinus thrombosis may present with eye pain. Raeder's paratrigeminal syndrome has many causes and is associated with eye pain. Horner's syndrome, often subtle, can be seen in carotidynia and carotid artery dissection. These conditions often present with pain radiating to the eye.

Acute angle closure glaucoma may mimic migraine or cluster headache. The headache is severe and unilateral with conjunctival injection. The pupil is usually mid-dilated and poorly reactive. "Protective ptosis" and a cloudy cornea may be present. The intraocular pressure is elevated during an attack. If one suspects this disorder, one should refer the patient to an ophthalmologist emergently.

Trochleitis and primary trochlear headache deserve special mention. The trochlea is a structure inside the medial canthus through which the tendon of the superior oblique muscle passes. Idiopathic trochleitis is a cause of superimposed ocular pain in patients with migraine. Trochleitis usually presents as orbital pain without obvious ocular signs. It may sustain or trigger the pain of chronic migraine. Diagnosis is confirmed by a peritrochlear steroid injection, which produces relief of periocular symptoms and may improve headache control. Orbital CT scan may show enlarged and asymmetrical trochlea. Patients with primary trochlear headache have pain in the trochlear area, without trochleitis or other orbital or systemic disease. Pain is exacerbated by direct palpation and supraduction of the eye. The temporal pattern is either chronic or remitting with acute exacerbations. About half of patients have increased pain at night. Many have concurrent headaches. Local injection of corticosteroids usually relieves the pain within 48 hours and often improves concurrent headache attack frequency. However, nearly half of patients relapse after an average of 8 months.

SINUS AND NASAL HEADACHE

The sinus and nasal areas can also be involved in producing or exacerbating headache. Acute rhinosinusitis develops rapidly and lasts from 1 day to 4 weeks. Characteristic symptoms include facial tenderness, pain, nasal congestion, and purulent discharge (Table 3.17). No single symptom is both sensitive and specific for sinusitis. Facial tenderness and pain, nasal congestion, anosmia, pain with mastication, halitosis, and a history of an upper respiratory infection are often present. Fever is present in half of patients, and headache is common, but these are of minimal value in diagnosing acute (or chronic) rhinosinusitis. The most specific symptom is maxillary toothache, but most patients do not have this symptom. A poor response to decongestants and the presence of pus or colored nasal discharge are diagnostically valuable. Pus may be absent in sphenoid sinusitis. Standard sinus x-rays are inadequate to evaluate rhinosinusitis. CT of the sinuses is necessary to define the anatomy before surgery and as a tool for management. CT or MRI is necessary to diagnose sphenoid sinusitis. Fiberoptic nasal endoscopy in combination with a negative neuroimaging study usually rules out sinus disease (Chapter 19).

TABLE 3.17 Sinusitis

- Acute rhinosinusitis
  - Sudden onset, lasts 1 day to 4 weeks
  - Facial tenderness and pain, nasal congestion, purulent discharge
  - Best predictors: maxillary toothache, abnormal transillumination, poor response to decongestants, purulent or colored nasal discharge
- Subacute, 4 to 12 weeks
- Chronic sinusitis, > 12 weeks—controversial
  - Headache continuous
  - Engorged or swollen mucosa
  - Purulent or bloody nasal discharge
- Nasal headache
  - Deviated septum
  - Bony septal spurs
  - Turbinate hypertrophy
  - Paradoxical turbinates
  - Concha bullosa

Nasal septal deviations, bony septal spurs, turbinate hypertrophy, paradoxical turbinates, and concha bullosa may cause nasal contact headache with symptoms that arise from the sinonasal region. The vast majority of these headaches are strictly or mostly unilateral. It is not clear how often these headaches are accompanied by migrainous features.

CERVICOGENIC HEADACHE

The cervical spine may produce or exacerbate headache. These headaches are usually unilateral without side shift, and are triggered by neck movements and certain postures; shoulder or arm pain and reduced range of motion are sometimes present. The pain is usually moderate, and may be episodic or continuous. Patients may have autonomic or migrainous symptoms. Their neck pain is often continuous. An anesthetic blockade that abolishes the pain may be necessary to make the diagnosis.

Migraineurs in particular are likely to have neck pain before, during, or after the headache. If we suspect that cervical disc disease is exacerbating headache, we look for interictal pain and neck symptoms and further test patients who have these. A differential diagnosis of cervical headaches is listed in Table 3.18.

Physical examination is of little value in diagnosing symptomatic joints, and diagnostic blocks are necessary. Myofascial pain may also cause neck pain radiating to the head. Physical examination and diagnostic trigger point injections are helpful, but paraspinal trigger point injections may also benefit migraine.

TABLE 3.18 Cervical Headache Differential

- Neck-tongue syndrome
- Lateral atlantoaxial joint pain
- Discogenic pain—C2–3 disc
- Zygoapophyseal (facet) pain (usually C2–3)
- Myofascial pain syndrome

TEETH AND MOUTH

Temporomandibular joint (TMJ) pain is usually intermittent and associated with use of the jaw. To diagnose TMJ, patients should display at least three of the following criteria: (1) limited range of motion, (2) joint noise, (3) tenderness to joint palpation, and (4) functional pain. Myofascial pain with referral to the head also occurs. Referred pain patterns usually do not make anatomic sense. Palpating the trigger point causes radiating pain that reproduces the patient's headache, and trigger point injections temporarily or permanently alleviate the pain.

HEADACHE BEGINNING IN LATE LIFE

Special attention is warranted when headaches begin late in life, because primary headaches rarely begin after the age of 50. Diagnostic testing (neuroimaging, erythrocyte sedimentation rate) is almost always indicated (Table 3.19).

TABLE 3.19 Common Causes of Headache Beginning in Late Life

Secondary headache disorders
- Mass lesions
- Giant cell arteritis
- Medication-related headache
- Trigeminal neuralgia (secondary)
- Postherpetic neuralgia
- Systemic disease
- Disease of the cranium, neck, eyes, ears, and nose
- Cerebrovascular disease
- Parkinson's disease

Primary headache disorders
- Migraine
- Tension-type headache
- Cluster headache
- Hypnic headache
- Trigeminal neuralgia (classical)

PRIMARY HEADACHE MISDIAGNOSIS

Sometimes one primary headache disorder is misdiagnosed as another. Hemicrania continua may be accompanied by the associated symptoms of migraine and may be misdiagnosed as chronic migraine or chronic daily headache. Chronic paroxysmal hemicrania may be mistaken for cluster headache; this may require an indomethacin trial to make the diagnosis. Hypnic headache may be misdiagnosed as cluster headache or chronic tension-type headache. Nummular headache can be mistaken for chronic tension-type headache.

At times, primary headaches take on symptoms that include the features of two different headaches: cluster-tic, migraine-tic, and cyclic migraine (which has both cluster and migraine features). See Chapter 15 for more details of unusual primary headache syndromes.

REFERENCES

ACOG Committee. Guidelines for diagnostic imaging during pregnancy. *Obstet Gynecol*. 2004;104:647–651.

Antonaci F, Ghirmai S, Bono G, Sandrini G, Nappi G. Cervicogenic headache: evaluation of the original diagnostic criteria. *Cephalalgia*. 2001;21:573–583.

Evans RW, Rozen TD, Mechtler L. Neuroimaging and other diagnostic testing in headache. In: Silberstein SD, Lipton RB, Dodick DW, eds. *Wolff's Headache and Other Head Pain*. 8th ed. New York, NY: Oxford University Press; 2008:63–93.

Kruit MC, vanBuchem MA, Hofman PA, et al. Migraine as a risk factor for subclinical brain lesions. *JAMA*. 2004;921:427–434.

Schwedt TJ, Matharu MS, Dodick DW. Thunderclap headache. *Lancet Neurol*. 2006;5:621–631.

Pathophysiology of Migraine and How to Explain It to Your Patients

INTRODUCTION

Headache is a pain syndrome involving the regions of the body innervated by the trigeminal and upper cervical nerves. Migraine is a primary headache disorder arising from brain dysfunction that may lead to activation of the trigeminal vascular system. Migraine is more than just a pain disorder—it also includes associated symptoms and multiple stages of an attack. The prodrome may begin as early as 3 days before an attack. Some patients have aura. The prodrome phase (and aura phase if present) is followed by the pain phase, which, when left untreated, can last from 4 to 72 hours.

ANATOMY OF HEADACHE

The fifth cranial nerve transmits all the somatic sensory information from the head, face, and dura to the trigeminal nucleus caudalis (TNC) in the central nervous system (CNS). The trigeminal nerve has three divisions: ophthalmic (first), mandibular (second), and maxillary (third). Anterior structures of the head and face are innervated by the ophthalmic division. Posterior regions of the head and neck are innervated by the upper cervical nerves. Trigeminal sensory neuron cell bodies are located in the trigeminal ganglion. A single neurite emerges from the cell bodies of the sensory neurons in the trigeminal ganglion, bifurcates, and projects out to the periphery and into the dorsal horn of the midbrain. Normally, we associate the direction of information transmission along this neuron from the periphery to the CNS, but glutamate and neuropeptides can also be released in the periphery. This can contribute to sensory trigeminal activation, blood vessel dilation, and plasma protein extravasation (Tables 4.1 and 4.2).

TABLE 4.1 Pain-sensitive Cranial Structures

- The scalp and its blood supply
- Parts of the dura mater
- Great venous sinuses
- Arteries of the meninges and larger cerebral vessels
- Pain-sensitive fibers of the fifth, ninth, and tenth cranial nerves

TABLE 4.2 What Causes Headaches?

- Traction, tension, or displacement of pain-sensitive structures
- Distention or dilation of intracranial arteries
- Inflammation of pain-sensitive structures
- Obstruction of CSF pathways with consequent increased intracranial pressure
- Primary central pain: involvement of pain-modulating systems

Abbreviation: CSF, cerebrospinal fluid.

AURA

Experts used to believe that the migraine aura was caused by cerebral vasoconstriction and the headache by reactive vasodilation. This theory explained the headache's throbbing quality and its relief by ergots. This vascular theory has been refuted, yet it continues to contaminate discussions of headache pathogenesis. It is now believed that the migraine aura is caused by neuronal dysfunction, not ischemia, and that ischemia rarely, if ever, occurs. Headache often begins when regional cerebral blood flow (rCBF) is reduced; thus, headache is not because of simple reflex vasodilation (Figure 4.1).

Migraine aura corresponds to a cortical event. Noxious stimulation of the rodent cerebral cortex produces a spreading increase and then decrease in electrical activity that moves at 2 to 3 mm/minute (cortical spreading depression [CSD]). CSD is characterized by shifts in cortical steady state potential, transient increases in potassium, nitric oxide, and glutamate, and transient increases in rCBF, followed by sustained decreases.

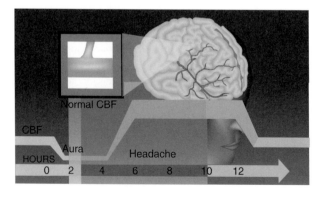

FIGURE 4.1 Cerebral blood flow (CBF) during a migraine attack. Blood flow is still decreased at headache onset.

Aura, CSD, and Spreading Oligemia

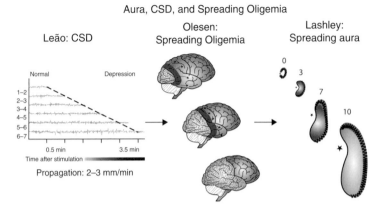

| Leão: CSD | Olesen: Spreading Oligemia | Lashley: Spreading aura |

FIGURE 4.2 Cortical spreading depression (CSD) results in spreading oligemia and spreading aura.
Source: Silberstein et al. *Headache in Clinical Practice* (2nd ed.). London: Martin; 2002.

The aura is associated with an initial hyperemic phase followed by reduced CBF, which moves across the cortex (spreading oligemia), usually posterior to anterior at 2 to 3 mm/minute. It crosses brain areas supplied by separate vessels, and is therefore not due to segmental vasoconstriction. Reduced rCBF persists for 30 minutes to 6 hours and then slowly returns to baseline or even above it. The rates of progression of spreading oligemia are similar to those of migraine aura and CSD, suggesting that these entities are related (Figure 4.2).

Magnetoencephalography demonstrates changes in migraineurs, but not controls, consistent with CSD. Using transcranial magnetic stimulation and applying magnetic fields of increasing intensity to evaluate occipital cortex excitability, researchers found that phosphenes were generated in migraineurs at lower thresholds than controls, and that it was easier to trigger headaches with visual stimuli in those with lower thresholds. Migraine with aura may be due to neuronal hyperexcitability, perhaps owing to cortical disinhibition.

HEADACHE

Headache probably results from activation of meningeal and blood vessel nociceptors combined with a change in central pain modulation. Headache and its associated neurovascular changes are subserved by the trigeminal system. Reflex connections to the cranial parasympathetics form the trigeminoautonomic reflex. Activation results in vasoactive intestinal polypeptide release and vasodilation.

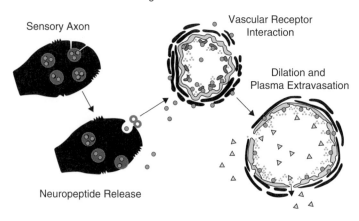

FIGURE 4.3 Neuropeptide release from sensory neurons results in blood vessel dilatation.

Trigeminal sensory neurons contain substance P (SP), calcitonin gene-related peptide (CGRP), and neurokinin A. Stimulation results in SP and CGRP release from sensory C-fiber terminals and neurogenic inflammation. The neuropeptides interact with the blood vessel wall, producing dilation, plasma protein extravasation, and platelet activation. Neurogenic inflammation sensitizes nerve fibers (peripheral sensitization) that now respond to previously innocuous stimuli, such as blood vessel pulsations, causing, in part, the pain of migraine. Central sensitization can also occur (Figure 4.3).

SENSITIZATION

Patients manifest sensory sensitization in two ways: hyperalgesia or allodynia. Hyperalgesia is present when slightly painful stimuli, such as a soft pinch, are perceived as very painful by the patient. During migraine attacks, patients complain of increased pain from stimuli that would ordinarily be non-nociceptive, a phenomenon called allodynia. These stimuli include brushing the hair, wearing a hat, showering, and resting the head on a pillow. As an attack progresses, many migraine sufferers develop cutaneous allodynia in the region of pain and then outside it at extracephalic locations (Table 4.3).

Sensitization of nociceptors, secondary sensory neurons in the TNC, or even the projection neurons in the thalamus are responsible for initiation and maintenance of the clinical symptoms of allodynia. Peripheral

TABLE 4.3 Migraine and Sensitization

- *Peripheral sensitization of trigeminovascular neurons*: mediates throbbing pain and its worsening by bending over
- *Central sensitization of trigeminovascular neurons in nucleus caudalis*: mediates scalp tenderness and increased periorbital skin sensitivity (i.e., cutaneous allodynia)
- *Allodynia*: nonpainful stimuli are painful

sensitization produces an increase in pain sensitivity that is restricted to the site of inflammation—in the case of migraine, this is the dura. This results in the throbbing quality of migraine pain and its activation by movement. Sensitization of these neurons reduces their threshold to a level where blood vessel and cerebrospinal fluid (CSF) pulsations are painful.

Patients often develop cutaneous allodynia during migraine attacks due to trigeminal sensitization. Triptans can prevent, but not reverse, cutaneous allodynia. Cutaneous allodynia can be used to predict triptans' effectiveness. In the absence of allodynia, triptans completely relieve the headache and block the development of allodynia. In 90% of attacks with established allodynia, triptans provide little or no headache relief and do not suppress allodynia. However, late triptan therapy eliminates peripheral sensitization (throbbing pain aggravated by movement) even when pain relief is incomplete and allodynia is not suppressed. Early intervention may work by preventing central sensitization.

Neuroimaging studies in primary headaches, such as migraine and cluster headache, have demonstrated activation in the brain areas associated with pain, such as the cingulate cortex, the insulae, the frontal cortex, the thalamus, the basal ganglia, and the cerebellum. These areas are similarly activated when head pain is induced by injecting capsaicin into volunteers' foreheads. In addition to the generic pain areas activated by the capsaicin injections, specific brainstem areas, such as the dorsal pons, are activated in episodic migraine. Patients with right-sided migraine headache showed increased rCBF in the left brainstem. Triptans relieve the headache and associated symptoms but do not normalize brainstem rCBF. This suggests that activation is because of factors other than, or in addition to, increased activity of the endogenous antinociceptive system.

PAIN MODULATION

The nervous system contains networks that modulate nociceptive transmission. The trigeminal brain stem nuclear complex receives monoaminergic, enkephalinergic, and peptidergic projections from regions that are important

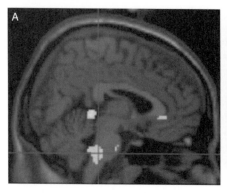 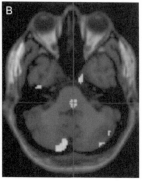

FIGURE 4.4 PET study exploring the laterality of brainstem activation in migraine using glyceryl trinitrate (GTN). Activation in migraine patients during a GTN-triggered migraine attack when compared with matched controls administered GTN in the same time course. (A) and (B) show activation in the dorsolateral pons, with anterior cingulate activation present in (A).

in the modulation of nociceptive systems. A descending inhibitory neuronal network extends from the frontal cortex and hypothalamus through the periaqueductal gray (PAG) to the rostral ventromedial medulla (RVM) and the medullary and spinal dorsal horn. The RVM includes the raphe nuclei and the adjacent reticular formation and projects to the outer laminae of the spinal and medullary dorsal horn. Electrical stimulation or injection of opioids into the PAG or RVM inhibits neuron activity in the dorsal horn. The PAG receives projections from the insular cortex and the amygdala (Figure 4.4). These nuclei are believed to modulate the activity of the TNC and the dorsal horn neurons. Three classes of neurons have been identified in the RVM and PAG.

"Off-cells" pause immediately before the nociceptive reflex, whereas "on-cells" are activated. Neutral cells show no consistent changes in activation. Increased on-cell activity in the brain stem pain modulation system enhances the response to both painful and nonpainful stimuli. Headache may be caused, in part, by enhanced neuronal activity in the TNC as a result of enhanced

TABLE 4.4 CNS Modulation of Migraine

- Brainstem aminergic nuclei can modify trigeminal pain processing
- Positron emission tomography demonstrates brainstem activation in spontaneous migraine attacks
- Brainstem activation persists after successful headache treatment
- Brainstem: generator or modulator

on-cell or decreased off-cell activity. Other conditioned stimuli associated with pain and stress also can turn on the pain system and may account, in part, for the association between pain and stress (Table 4.4).

GENETICS

Migraine is a group of familial disorders with a genetic component. Familial hemiplegic migraine (FHM) is an autosomal dominant disorder associated with attacks of migraine, with and without aura, and hemiparesis. The gene has been mapped to chromosome 19p13 in approximately two thirds of cases. The defect is due to at least 10 different missense mutations in the CACNA1A gene, which codes for the α1-subunit of a voltage-dependent P/Q Ca^{2+} channel. P-type neuronal Ca^{2+} channels mediate serotonin (5-HT) and excitatory neurotransmitter release. Dysfunction may impair 5-HT release and predispose patients to migraine attacks or impair their self-aborting mechanism. Voltage-gated P/Q-type calcium channels mediate glutamate release, are involved in CSD, and may be integral to initiation of the migraine aura. A second gene (FHM2) has been mapped to chromosome 1q21–23. The defect is a new mutation in the α2-subunit of the Na^+/K^+ pump resulting in reduced activity or decreased affinity for K+ of Na^+/K^+ pump leading to impaired clearance of K^+ and glutamate from the extracellular space. A third gene (FHM3) has been linked to chromosome 2q24. It is because of a missense mutation in gene SCN1A (Gln1489Lys), which encodes an α1-subunit of a neuronal voltage-gated Na^+ channel (Nav1.1). This results in a 2- to 4-fold accelerated recovery from fast inactivation and results in excessive firing of neurons. This could facilitate CSD by several mechanisms. Repetitive firing might enhance the release of the excitatory neurotransmitter glutamate. This mutation might have effects similar to those of CACNA1A mutations in FHM1, which enhance neurotransmitter release and facilitate CSD. This is also similar to the effects of the ATP1A2 mutations in FHM2 (Table 4.5).

TABLE 4.5 Genetic Basis

Twin studies: monozygotic > dizygotic
FHM
■ FHM1 (19p13): *CACNA1A* encodes α_1-subunit of voltage-gated neuronal $Ca_v2.1$(P/Q) Ca^{2+} channel: 50% of cases
■ FHM2 (1q23): *ATP1A2* encodes α_2-subunit of Na^+/K^+ pump
■ FHM3 (2q24): SCN1A encodes α_1-subunit of neuronal voltage-gated Na^+ channel $Na_v1.1$

Abbreviation: FHM, familial hemiplegic migraine.

HOW TO EXPLAIN THIS TO PATIENTS

It is important for patients with migraine to understand they have a primary neurobiological condition. Too often they are led to believe, either by laypeople, popular culture, or even other physicians, that they are crazy, overstressed, or have something ominous, like a brain tumor. Some patients even think it is their own fault somehow that they get migraines. Emphasize certain points, using terms the patient can understand, when explaining the biological basis for migraine.

1. Migraine is a disorder of a sensitive brain. Patients are more sensitive to light, sound, and other stimuli than usual, both during and between attacks. Certain stimuli (e.g., lights, visual patterns, odors, foods, or other substances) and disruptions of the natural biological balance (e.g., unanticipated stress, changes in sleep habits or dietary patterns) often trigger migraines.

2. Definite changes happen in the brain and blood vessels before, during, and after migraine attacks. Waves of reduced brain activity and blood flow sweep over the brain surface, corresponding to many of the nonpain features of migraine. Blood vessels constrict and dilate at different stages of the attack. Chemicals that make certain structures even more sensitive are released, resulting in increased pain.

3. Having migraines does not mean you are crazy. It is true that many patients with uncontrolled headaches become depressed, and many patients with depression also have migraines. It is true that mood disturbances can trigger headaches. It is true that antidepressants are often used to treat migraines because there is some common ground between the two in terms of the neurochemical imbalances that underlie each. It is not true that migraines and mental problems directly cause one another.

4. The reason migraine medications work is that they affect one or more of the biological processes that occur in patients with migraine, both during and between attacks.

5. There is a genetic basis for migraine, which is further evidence that this is a "real" disorder. Although there is no one specific gene for it, migraine and related conditions often run in families. Specific genes are connected to certain rare types of migraine, like hemiplegic migraine (these patients become paralyzed on one side during attacks), and these genes are responsible for dysfunction of the neuron channels that regulate chemical balances.

6. Although headaches sometimes indicate that something serious is going on, in most cases they are a primary neurologic problem. When symptoms are consistent with what most other people experience with migraine, the examination is normal, typical medications work like they are supposed to,

and no "red flags" are present in the history, we are very confident that the patient has primary migraine.

7. It is not your fault that you have migraines, but there are things that you do every day that can either help or hurt you as you learn to live with the problem. Keeping everything in your life as balanced and healthful as possible is important in maintaining control. Of course, following your doctor's advice at all times is also extremely important.

CONCLUSION

The migraine aura is probably due to CSD. Headache probably results from activation of meningeal and blood vessel nociceptors combined with a change in central pain modulation. Headache and its associated neurovascular changes are subserved by the trigeminal system. Stimulation results in the release of SP and CGRP from sensory C-fiber terminals and neurogenic inflammation. Neurogenic inflammation sensitizes nerve fibers (peripheral sensitization), which now respond to previously innocuous stimuli, such as blood vessel pulsations, causing, in part, the pain of migraine. Central sensitization of TNC neurons can also occur. Central sensitization may play a key role in maintaining the headache. Brainstem activation also occurs in migraine without aura, in part because of increased activity of the endogenous antinociceptive system. The migraine aura can trigger headache: CSD activates trigeminovascular afferents. Stress can also activate meningeal plasma cells via a parasympathetic mechanism, leading to nociceptor activation.

REFERENCES

Afridi SK, Matharu MS, Lee L, et al. A PET study exploring the laterality of brainstem activation in migraine using glyceryl trinitrate. *Brain*. 2005:128; 932–939.

Charles A. Advances in the basic and clinical science of migraine. *Ann Neurol.* 2009;65(5):491–498.

Ferrari MD, Dichgans M. Genetics of primary headache. In: Silberstein SD, Lipton RB, Dodick DW, eds. *Wolff's headache and Other Head Pain.* 8th ed. New York, NY: Oxford University Press; 2008:133–152.

Goadsby PJ, Oshinsky ML. Pathophysiology of headache. In: Silberstein SD, Lipton RB, Dodick DW, eds. *Wolff's Headache and Other Head Pain.* 8th ed. New York., NY: Oxford University Press; 2008:105–120.

Olesen J, Burstein R, Ashina M, Tfelt-Hansen P. Origin of pain in migraine: evidence for peripheral sensitization. *Lancet Neurol.* 2009;8(7):679–690.

5 Migraine: Treating the Acute Attack

Migraine headache is a highly disabling neurologic disease that usually requires prescription medication for acute attacks. In addition to pain, migraine is associated with nausea (with or without vomiting) and light and sound sensitivity. Other symptoms include neck pain, congestion or sinus pressure, and fatigue. The goals of acute treatment are to reduce pain and suffering, alleviate coexisting symptoms, and reduce disability. All patients need to have a specific acute treatment plan in place (Table 5.1).

TABLE 5.1 Principles of Acute Treatment for Episodic Migraine

- Use acute treatment to reduce pain, disability, and/or suffering
- Individualize treatment
- Treat early in the attack with adequate dosing
- Monitor prescription and over-the-counter acute medication use
- Consider nonoral medications when nausea or vomiting is present
- Include a rescue treatment

THE BASICS OF ACUTE MIGRAINE TREATMENT

Stratified Care

Two basic strategies, step care and stratified care, are used to treat acute migraine. In the step-care model, patients progress through a sequence of medications—usually starting with a simple analgesic, then perhaps an antiemetic, and then a specific medication if the initial treatments are ineffective. This can mean escalating treatment across or within attacks. With stratified care, attacks are treated based on severity. In this model, patients use nonspecific medications for minimally disabling attacks and specific medications for severe attacks. Stratified care improves treatment outcomes, improves quality of life, and reduces costs (Table 5.2).

Treat Early

Treating migraine with specific medication early in the attack improves outcomes. Patients who take triptans early, when the pain is still mild, have increased pain-free rates. When taken early, triptans may prevent the development of central sensitization, as manifested clinically by cutaneous allodynia

TABLE 5.2 Step Care and Stratified Care

Step Care	Stratified Care
■ Start with simple analgesic (i.e., acetaminophen, NSAID) ■ If not effective, take second line medication (such as an antiemetic) ■ If initial treatments fail, use specific medication	■ Treat attacks based on attack severity ■ Use simple analgesics for mild attacks ■ Use specific medication early for severe attacks

Abbreviation: NSAID, nonsteroidal anti-inflammatory drug.

(pain in response to normally nonpainful stimuli). Once cutaneous allodynia has developed, patients are less likely to respond to triptans.

Monitor Frequency of Medication Use

Overuse of acute pain medication is a complication of frequent headache and can lead to increased headache frequency and treatment refractoriness. Medication overuse headache (MOH) is defined as using simple analgesics more than 15 days a month or using triptans, ergots, opioids, or combination medications more than 10 days a month for more than 3 months. There is no credit for using multiple abortive types if the patient still uses any abortive more than one-half of the days of the month.

MOH affects migraine patients more than patients with other headache disorders and is one cause of chronic daily headache (CDH). Treating MOH by withdrawing the offending agent can bring about improvement, but often only after a period of increased headache that lasts days to weeks to months. Migraineurs should be aware of MOH and keep a calendar or diary of their headaches and acute medication use. MOH can also cause adverse events (AEs), such as ergotism, constipation, gastrointestinal and renal disease, or tardive dyskinesias, specific to the class of medication (Table 5.3).

It is difficult for patients with frequent headaches or CDH to avoid medication overuse. To manage this risk and navigate between undertreatment and medication overuse, we use "the rule of 4s": If headache days are <4 per month, be aggressive in treating every migraine. In general, treat aggressively; however, some restraint is indicated, and if headache frequency is >8 per month, stress the use of preventive treatment, coping, nonsteroidal anti-inflammatory drugs (NSAIDs), and neuroleptics, and modify the early treatment paradigm.

Individualize Treatment

When selecting acute migraine medication, individualize the treatment according to the headache's characteristics. For rapidly escalating, disabling

TABLE 5.3 Consequences of Medicine Overuse—Common AEs by Class

Drug Class	AEs
Triptans	CDH, increased vascular risk?
Ergots	Muscle cramps, ergotism (gangrene), nausea, fibrotic disorders, CDH
NSAIDs	Ulcers, renal disease, easy bruising
Opioids	Constipation, dependence, addiction, CDH
Barbiturates	Sedation, dependence, CDH
Neuroleptics/antiemetics	Sedation, weight gain, tardive dyskinesias, parkinsonism

Abbreviations: AEs, adverse events; CDH, chronic daily headache; NSAIDs, nonsteroidal anti-inflammatory drugs.

attacks, consider injectable medications. Patients with significant nausea or vomiting should use non-oral medications and antiemetics. Before deciding that a treatment is ineffective, patients should treat at least two attacks. Other strategies include changing the dose, using a different formulation or route of administration, or adding a second agent.

Include a Rescue Medication

Migraineurs need a rescue treatment for attacks that do not respond to specific medication and require frequent, urgent physician or emergency room visits. In most cases, rescue medications do not eliminate pain or allow normal functioning. Many rescue treatments, such as neuroleptics, corticosteroids, or opioids, may cause sedation but can provide some relief and help avoid an emergency room visit. Frequent migraines or those that do not respond to acute agents indicate that migraine prevention is probably warranted.

Medications

Acute attack medications include those specific for migraine (and cluster) headache, such as triptans, ergots and dihydroergotamine (DHE), and nonspecific medications (those used for headache and other pain disorders) (Table 5.4).

Specific medications
Triptans
Triptans are selective serotonin receptor agonists with high affinity for 5-HT$_{1B}$ and 5-HT$_{1D}$ receptors and variable activity at the 5-HT$_{1F}$ receptor. Although initial research suggested that the effectiveness of triptans occurred because of their vasoconstrictive properties, their ability to both block the transmission of pain signals from the trigeminal nerve to the trigeminal nucleus caudalis and

TABLE 5.4 Combination Medications Containing Caffeine and/or Butalbital

Specific Medications	Nonspecific Medications
Triptans	Nonsteroidal anti-inflammatory drugs (NSAIDs)
Ergotamine	Antiemetics/neuroleptics
DHE	Opioids
	Combination medications containing caffeine and butalbital
	Corticosteroids

Abbreviations: DHE, dihydroergotamine; NSAIDs, nonsteroidal anti-inflammatory drugs.

prevent release of inflammatory neuropeptides is more important. Triptans are well tolerated and effective, with an excellent safety profile and without the risk of dependence or addiction seen with butalbital or opioid medications. Currently seven different triptans are available for migraine. Each triptan has different pharmacologic properties; some are available in different formulations, such as orally disintegrating tablets, nasal sprays (NS), or subcutaneous injection (SC) (Table 5.5).

Triptan choice depends on the patient's headache patterns, how medications are metabolized, and what AEs are experienced (Table 5.6). SC sumatriptan is the most effective and fastest-acting triptan, but it causes the most AEs. A meta-analysis of 53 trials evaluating oral triptans compared all oral triptans to sumatriptan 100 mg. Rizatriptan 10 mg had better efficacy and consistency. Eletriptan 80 mg had better efficacy but more AEs and more potential drug interactions. Furthermore, this dose is not available and it may only be given once in 24 hours. Almotriptan 12.5 mg had better pain-free response and fewer AEs. Naratriptan 2.5 mg, frovatriptan 2.5 mg, and sumatriptan 25 mg had lower response rates at 2 hours, but naratriptan 2.5 mg and sumatriptan 25 mg were better tolerated than sumatriptan 100 mg. Zolmitriptan 2.5 and 5 mg, rizatriptan 5 mg, and eletriptan 40 mg had similar results compared with sumatriptan 100 mg. In clinical practice, patients vary in their characteristics and response patterns. Trial and error is often necessary to find the best treatment. If one triptan fails, it is worth trying another.

Sumatriptan is now available in combination with naproxen. This sequential time-release formulation decreases headache recurrence and is more effective for migraine than either sumatriptan or naproxen alone.

For simplicity, we dose all triptans in the following manner: take one as needed for migraine, may repeat in 2 hours, and limit to 2 per day, 2 days a week. Exceptions include frovatriptan (which may be repeated in 4 hours), rizatriptan (max 24-hour dose, 30 mg), and ½ dose tablets (could take more tablets per 24 hours).

TABLE 5.5 Serotonin 5-HT$_{1B/1D}$ Agonists (Triptans)

Medication	Formulations	Doses (mg)	Tmax (hours)	Half-life (hours)	Comments
Almotriptan	po	6.25, 12.5	2.1	3.1	Best side effects profile with good efficacy
Eletriptan	po	20, 40	1.8	5	80 mg dose is safe but more side effects and not approved in USA
Frovatriptan	po	2.5	~2.5	~26	Also used in miniprophylaxis of menstrually-related migraine
Naratriptan	po	1, 2.5	2	6	
Rizatriptan	po, tablet or dissolvable (ODT)	5[a], 10	2–3	2	Perhaps most effective oral formulation
Sumatriptan	po	25, 50, 100	1.5	2	Now generic
	NS	20	1.5	1.8	Bad taste
	SC	4, 6	0.17	2	Most effective way to give triptan
Sumatriptan/ naproxen	po	85/500			Only 1 of 3 will take separate pills simultaneously if prescribed as single treatment
Zolmitriptan	po, tablet or ODT	2.5, 5	3	3	
Zolmitriptan	NS	5	3	3	More effective; better taste than sumatriptan NS

Abbreviations: NS, nasal sprays; ODT, orally disintegrating tablets; po, oral.

[a] Use the 5-mg dose in patients taking propranolol.

TABLE 5.6 Choosing a Triptan

Clinical Situation	Triptan(s) of Choice
Rapidly escalating, severe attacks	Sumatriptan SC 4 or 6 mg, zolmitriptan NS 5 mg
Can't swallow, severe nausea	Sumatriptan SC 4 or 6 mg, zolmitriptan NS 5 mg, sumatriptan NS 20 mg, rizatriptan ODT 5 or 10 mg, zolmitriptan ODT 2.5 or 5 mg
Severe attacks (in patients preferring oral triptans)	Rizatriptan 10 mg, eletriptan 40 mg, sumatriptan/naproxen 85 mg/500 mg
Patient taking monoamine-oxidase inhibitors (MAO-I)	Eletriptan 20 or 40 mg, frovatriptan 2.5 mg, naratriptan 1 or 2.5 mg
Triptans poorly tolerated	Almotriptan 6.25 or 12.5 mg, naratriptan 2.5 mg, sumatriptan 25 mg

Abbreviations: NS, nasal spray; SC, subcutaneous; ODT, orally disintegrating tablet.

Common triptan-related AEs include paresthesias, dizziness, weakness, nausea, and fatigue. Transient throat and chest tightness may occur but are rarely related to coronary artery disease. Because of their potential for vasoconstriction, triptans are contraindicated for patients with ischemic heart disease, vasospasm, uncontrolled hypertension, or transient ischemic attacks. There have been reports of possible serotonin syndrome in patients taking both triptans and selective serotonin reuptake inhibitors (SSRIs) or other antidepressants. However, headache specialists are convinced that the FDA was unjustified in issuing a black box warning for serotonin syndrome when combining SSRIs or serotonin-norepinephrine reuptake inhibitors (SNRI) and triptans. The cases cited as serotonin syndrome because of this combination do not actually fulfill the criteria for the phenomenon. Furthermore, serotonin syndrome is mediated by the 5-HT_{2A} receptor, for which triptans have no affinity; so it is not even plausible that serotonin syndrome could occur with this combination. Despite this, rumors continue to fly freely, and pharmacists continue to refuse to fill triptan prescriptions for individuals on certain antidepressants. Do your best to educate them!

Ergotamine and DHE

Ergotamine and DHE (an ergot derivative) are older medications for moderate to severe migraine. Both are serotonin agonists with vasoconstrictive and α-adrenergic activity. Ergotamine has more arterial vasoconstriction than DHE, which is a more potent α-adrenergic antagonist with less emetic effect. Ergotamine causes more AEs, especially nausea and vomiting, than triptans, which limits its usefulness. Ergotamine is available as suppositories or tablets with and without caffeine. DHE

TABLE 5.7 Ergotamine and DHE

Drug	Dose	Route
Ergotamine	1 or 2 mg	Oral
		Suppository
Ergotamine and caffeine	1 mg/100 mg	Oral
DHE	2 mg	NS
	1 mg	IM, IV, SC
	1 mg	Inhaled

Abbreviations: DHE, dihydroergotamine; IM, intramuscular; IV, intravenous; SC, subcutaneous.

is available as NS and SC, intramuscular (IM), and intravenous (IV) injection. Nausea is less common with the NS, SC, and IM forms of DHE than with IV treatment. To avoid the nausea, administer an antiemetic before giving IV DHE. DHE is particularly useful for patients with frequent, severe migraine and may be less likely to produce MOH than ergots or triptans. Like triptans, DHE and ergots should not be used for patients with coronary or cerebral vascular disease. They are also contraindicated for those with uncontrolled hypertension, sepsis, pregnancy, and renal or hepatic failure. An inhaled form of DHE (Levadex) has blood levels similar to IV DHE without the immediate spike (first 3 minutes) responsible for the nausea and most of the chest symptoms (Table 5.7).

Nonspecific medications
Despite the emergence of triptans, nonspecific medications are still popular, and triptans are still underutilized. Few direct comparisons of specific and nonspecific medications exist, and some patients may find combinations of nonspecific medications to be superior. Because many patients have contraindications to specific agents, and because they are not always effective or well tolerated, clinicians should be comfortable prescribing multiple classes of nonspecific medications for acute migraine.

Nonsteroidal anti-inflammatory drugs
NSAIDs are effective for the acute treatment of migraine. They may work by suppressing inflammation and by preventing and treating central sensitization by blocking glial production of prostaglandins. They may also treat other migraine symptoms, such as neck pain and sinus pressure, that are commonly associated with acute migraine attacks. NSAIDs are less likely to cause MOH than other treatments, but their frequent use can lead to systemic AEs, such as peptic ulcers or renal disease. NSAIDs that have proven effectiveness in migraine (Table 5.8) can be combined with triptans and antiemetics for severe attacks.

TABLE 5.8 Nonsteroidal Anti-inflammatory Drugs

Drug	Route	Dose (mg)	Frequency
Carboxylic acids			
Salicylates			
Aspirin	po	325–1000	tid-qid (max 4000 mg)
Diflunisal (Dolobid)	po	250–1000	tid (max 1500 mg)
Salsalate (Disalcid)	po	500–1500	bid
Choline magnesium			
trisalicylate (Trilisate)	po	500–1500	bid
Acetic acid derivatives			
Diclofenac			bid-tid
(Voltaren, Cataflam)	po	25–75	(max 150 mg)
Etodolac (Lodine)	po	200–500	qid (max 1000 mg)
Tolmetin (Tolectin)	po	200–600	tid
Sulindac (Clinoril)	po	150–200	bid
Indomethacin (Indocin)	po	25–75	tid-qid (max 300 mg)
	PR	50	tid-qid
	IM/IV[a]	50	tid-qid
Propionic acids			
Ibuprofen			
(Motrin, Advil)	po	200–800	tid
Ketoprofen (Orudis)	po	50	tid
Fenoprofen (Nalfon)	po	200–600	qid
Flurbiprofen (Ansaid)	po	50–100	tid
Naproxen			bid-tid
(Aleve, Anaprox)	po	500–1100	(max max 1650 mg)
Ketorolac (Toradol)	po	10	tid
	IM	30–60	bid
	IV	15–30	tid-qid
Oxaprozin (Daypro)	po	600	tid
Fenamic acids			
Mefanemic acid			
(Ponstel)	po	250–500	qid (max 1000 mg)
Meclofenamate			
(Meclomen)	po	50–100	qid
Enolic acids (Oxicams)			
Meloxicam (Mobic)	po	7.5–15	daily
Piroxicam (Feldene)	po	10	bid
Nonacidic			
Celecoxib (Celebrex)	po	100–400	bid
Nabumetone (Relafen)	po	500–750	tid (max 1500 mg)

Abbreviations: IM, intramuscular; IV, intravenous; po, oral; PR, suppository.

[a] Not available in US.

TABLE 5.9 Half-lives of NSAIDs

Short	Intermediate	Long
Salicylates (except diflunisal)	Diflunisal	Oxaprozin
Profens (except flurbiprofen)	Flurbiprofen	Nabumetone
Fenamic acids	Naproxen	Meloxicam
Ketorolac	Sulindac	Piroxicam (longest)
Diclofenac	Etodolac	
Indomethacin	Celecoxib	
Tolmetin		

Abbreviation: NSAIDs, nonsteroidal anti-inflammatory drugs.

Most NSAIDs have a short or intermediate half-life, but a few have long half-lives. Shorter half-life drugs may have shorter duration AEs, and longer half-life drugs might have more utility in long-lasting or recurrent headaches, but neither of these concepts is truly a general rule (Table 5.9).

Since some AEs associated with NSAIDs are because of COX-1 inhibition, selective COX-2 inhibitors were developed. Currently, only one of these engineered drugs remains available, due to the demonstrated cardiac risk of long-term use in susceptible individuals. However, some of the older NSAIDs actually have some COX-2 selectivity (Table 5.10).

Opioids

Opioids provide therapeutic benefit but are associated with a high risk of abuse, dependency, and MOH. Opioids are most useful for patients with infrequent

TABLE 5.10 COX-2 selectivity of NSAIDs

<5x COX-2	5–50x COX-2	>50x COX-2
Fenoprofen	Etodolac	Lumaricoxib (in development)
Ibuprofen	Diclofenac	Etoricoxib (in development)
Tolmetin	Celecoxib	Rofecoxib (withdrawn)
Naproxen	Meloxicam	Veldecoxib (withdrawn)
Aspirin		
Indomethacin		
Ketoprofen		
Flurbiprofen		
Ketorolac		

Abbreviation: NSAIDs, nonsteroidal anti-inflammatory drugs.

Going down each list, COX-2 selectivity diminishes. Ketorolac has >50x COX-1 selectivity.

but disabling migraine, especially if a patient has contraindications (such as cardiovascular disease or pregnancy) to specific treatments. Although AEs may include sedation or confusion, patients might use opioids as a rescue medication to avoid a visit to the emergency room. Codeine with acetaminophen is effective in migraine, and other opioids commonly used as rescue treatments include fentanyl, hydromorphone, hydrocodone, methadone, morphine, oxycodone, propoxyphene, and pentazocine. Meperidine IM and IV is commonly used but may cause AEs, such as seizures. The agonist-antagonist opioid butorphanol has lower abuse potential (in theory) and can be given IV (2–3 mg) or as a NS.

Treating frequent migraine with opioids is problematic and should be considered only under certain circumstances. Do not use opioids when patients have addictive tendencies, a history of substance abuse, severe psychiatric disorders, or MO. Fewer than 20% of patients taking long-term daily opioids for CDH have sustained improvement, and many patients are nonadherent. When using opioids, prescribe with strict limits and monitor the patient closely (Table 5.11).

TABLE 5.11 Proposed Guidelines for Continuous Opioid Therapy for Refractory Chronic Daily Headache: Patient Selection Criteria and Formal Treatment Monitoring Requirements

A. All of the following (1–5) are required
1. The patient is an adult over age 30
2. Moderate to severe, convincing pain and functional compromise occur more than 20 days/month
3. A history of reliable and compliant medication usage and related behavior
4. At least four clinical visits with prescribing physicians over several months' time with personal, direct treatment encounters prior to opioid administration. (Physicians must know the patient and have a reasonable understanding of the level of intractability, compliance, maturity, and psychological makeup)
5. The prescribing physician has competence, knowledge, and experience in the use of the scheduled opioid

B. At least one of the following (1–5) must also apply
1. Convincing refractoriness to aggressive, advanced, comprehensive treatment, which should include the following:
   a. Ruling out and treating MOH (if present)
   b. Appropriately aggressive pharmacotherapy
   c. Cognitive-behavioral pain management
   d. Interventional treatment, if indicated
   e. Diagnostic review to rule out organic and pathological disturbances
2. The presence of convincing, serious AEs from otherwise appropriate medications, severely limiting available treatments

TABLE 5.11 Proposed Guidelines for Continuous Opioid Therapy (*Continued*)

3. Senior individual (e.g., >65 years old) for whom other treatments are ineffective or pose safety concerns. (Note that relative risk of respiratory depression rises significantly with age, and that seniors may reach efficacy with significantly lower doses)
4. Individual with significant medical comorbidities for whom other options for treatment are not available or contraindicated
5. Pregnancy, in which other acceptable treatments are ineffective and pain control is required (Note possible developmental delay with sustained opioids—coordinate care with patient's obstetrician)

C. Any of the following (1–6) would generally disqualify
1. Severe Axis I DSM-IV diagnosis, or multiple diagnoses of moderate severity (exception—some patients with mood disorders attributed to their medical condition may experience significant improvement in depression with pain relief)
2. Past or present true addictive disease (exception—nondrinking, rehabilitated alcoholic)
3. Axis II Cluster B personality disorders (significant antisocial, borderline, histrionic, or narcissistic traits)
4. Presence of moderate to severe somatoform features
5. Active psychosis or Axis II Cluster A personality disorders (paranoid, schizoid, schizotypal)
6. Known substance abuser in family environment (exception—history of long-term sustained remission following treatment participation)

D. A formal treatment monitoring system for appropriate use, safety, efficacy, and functional effect must be in place
1. Written, signed, and witnessed pretreatment agreement
   a. Compliance expectations
   b. Collateral discussions with family member or significant other
   c. Collateral discussions with other treatment professionals
   d. Agreement and plan for safe withdrawal from COT in the event that the prescribing physician or patient believes that discontinuation is in patient's best interest
2. Pretreatment and ongoing urine drug screens
3. Regular office visits every 1 to 2 months, including periodic contact with family members or significant others to assess efficacy, functioning, and adverse effects
4. Periodic psychological consultation to assess compliance, efficacy, functioning, psychological benefit or AEs, adherence to self-help and cognitive-behavioral pain management techniques
5. Calculation of dose and pill counts coordinated with frequency of visits
6. Formal assessment of efficacy and functional effect at each visit
7. Periodic communication with all treating professionals
8. Pretreatment and periodic updates (through state registries, when available) of all scheduled drugs that a patient has been prescribed and filled in the past year

Abbreviations: AEs, adverse events; COT, continuous opioid therapy; DSM-IV-TR, Diagnostic and Statistical Manual of Mental Disorders, Fourth Edition, Text Revision; MOH, medication overuse headache.

TABLE 5.12 Risks for Aberrant Drug-related Behavior

- Family history of substance abuse
- Personal history of substance abuse
- Younger age
- History of preadolescent sexual abuse
- Psychiatric disease
- Male gender

TABLE 5.13 Behaviors Associated with Opioid Treatment

Probably Aberrant	Probably Not Aberrant
- Selling, forging, stealing, and borrowing - Injecting orals - Buying on street - Concurrent illicits - Multiple unauthorized dose escalations - Losing scripts	- Aggressively complaining for more - Hoarding when feeling well - Specific requests - Multisourcing - Dose escalation 1–2x - Using for other symptoms

Patients should sign a consent and treatment agreement that outlines the risks and benefits of treatment and outlines expectations with adherence to the treatment plan.

Perform drug screening prior to initiation of opioids. If drugs associated with abuse are present, do not prescribe opioids until this situation is remedied. Thereafter, perform random drug screening. Optimally, use a service that will provide quantitative results with an analysis of drug levels and metabolites that can verify whether a patient is taking medications as prescribed. Screen and monitor patients for aberrant drug-related behaviors. Patients at high risk, and those who display aberrant behaviors, require closer monitoring and perhaps should be withdrawn from or denied opioid treatment. Patients must not receive opioid prescriptions from multiple providers (Tables 5.12 and 5.13).

Barbiturates

Butalbital-containing analgesics include combinations of acetaminophen or aspirin with caffeine and, sometimes, codeine. No clinical trial has demonstrated that butalbital, a barbiturate, adds to the effectiveness of the constituent components, and the risk of dependency and MOH is high. As with opioids, butalbital-containing medication use must be monitored closely and limited to situations wherein other treatments are ineffective or contraindicated.

Antiemetics and neuroleptics

Neuroleptics are antidopaminergic medications that block dopamine at D2 receptors in the brain. They are usually effective both for treating pain and improving the nausea or vomiting associated with migraine. Neuroleptics are often effective even in severe migraine and many are available as PR, IM, or IV treatments (Table 5.14). They are effective as rescue medications, and studies suggest that neuroleptics are underutilized in the emergency room for the treatment of acute migraine. Other antiemetics work by antagonizing serotonin 5-HT$_3$ receptors.

Oral metoclopramide is effective as an adjuvant medication with NSAIDs or triptans and decreases gastric stasis that can impair absorption of medications. Chlorpromazine, droperidol, prochlorperazine, and haloperidol are all useful for acute migraine, including refractory cases. Sedation and extrapyramidal AEs are common. Promethazine and hydroxyzine are antiemetics that are less likely to cause extrapyramidal AEs. Serotonin receptor (5-HT$_3$) antagonists may help treat nausea but do not appear effective for migraine pain (Table 5.14). All neuroleptics, except for metoclopramide, can cause prolongation of the QTc interval and should be avoided in patients with this problem (>450 ms for men and >460 ms for women). Check EKG prior to starting neuroleptic treatment, and monitor EKGs in actively treated patients.

TABLE 5.14 Neuroleptics for Migraine

Drug	Route	Dose (mg)	Frequency
Metoclopramide (Reglan)	po	5–10	tid-qid
	IM	10	tid-qid
	IV	10–20	tid-qid
Prochlorperazine (Compazine)	po	5–10	tid-qid
	PR	25	tid-qid
	IV	5–10	tid-qid
Promethazine (Phenergan)	po	10	tid-qid
	PR	25	tid-qid
	po	12.5–100	Hourly until relief or sleep
Chlorpromazine (Thorazine)	IV	12.5–100	tid-qid
Droperidol (Inapsine)	IM	2.5	tid-qid (max 10 mg)
	IV	0.625–2.5	tid-qid (max 10 mg)
Haloperidol (Haldol)	po	2–10	tid-qid
	IV	1–10	tid-qid
Olanzapine (Zyprexa)	po	2.5–20	hourly until relief or sleep, max 20 mg

Abbreviations: IM, intramuscular; IV, intravenous; po, oral; PR, suppository.

TABLE 5.15 Other Oral Analgesics for Migraine

Drug	Dose
Acetaminophen	325–1000 mg
Isometheptene mucate/dichloralphenazone/ acetaminophen (Midrin)	65 mg/100 mg/325 mg
Acetaminophen/aspirin/caffeine (Excedrin)	250 mg/250 mg/65 mg
Acetaminophen/isometheptene/caffeine (Migraten)	325 mg/100 mg/65 mg

Other analgesics

Acetaminophen is effective for migraine at a dose of 1000 mg and is useful for patients with contraindications to NSAIDs. Caffeine enhances the effect of other migraine medications and has analgesic properties of its own. Acetaminophen and caffeine are often used in combination medications. The combination of isometheptene (a sympathomimetic), dichloralphenazone (a choral hydrate derivative), and acetaminophen is modestly effective and relatively well tolerated (this is marketed under the trade name Midrin; a similar drug marketed under the name Migraten substitutes caffeine for dichloralphenazone). Contraindications include glaucoma, renal failure, severe hypertension, heart or renal disease, and monoamine-oxidase inhibitors (MAO-I) (Table 5.15).

Prodrome and aura

Treating migraine when premonitory symptoms, such as hunger, neck pain, thirst, or drowsiness, are present, before the headache begins, is occasionally effective. Domperidone 20 to 40 mg and metoclopramide may help prevent headaches, and triptans also may be useful. No medication is proven to reverse the neuronal dysfunction of prolonged migraine aura, but case reports suggest IV magnesium 1000 mg, ketamine NS 25 mg, and carbon dioxide may be effective. Transcranial magnetic stimulation is effective for some patients in experimental studies.

Bridge therapy

Bridges are treatments given for an intermediate length of time, usually 3 to 7 days, for status migrainosus or exacerbations of chronic migraine (Table 5.16). They are often useful when the goal is stopping overused medications (triptans, combination drugs, or opioids) before preventive treatments become effective. Steroids are often effective for this, as are combinations of NSAIDs and an antiemetic. Our goal is to keep the patient functional and avoid IV treatments or hospital admission; so advise a higher dose of antiemetics before bedtime.

TABLE 5.16 Bridge Therapy

Steroids	Dose	Example Instructions
Methylprednisolone	1 dose pack	Use as directed (6 days)
Prednisone	Start 60–80 mg, decrease over 3–6 days	20 mg, 3po day 1–2; 2 po day 3–4, 1 po day 5–6
Dexamethasone	Decrease over 3–6 days	4 mg, 3 for day 1, 2 for day 2, and 1 for day 3
NSAIDs		
Naproxen sodium	550 mg tid	550 tid × 5 days
Nabumetone + metoclopramide	550 mg + 10 mg over 3–7 days	550 mg + 10 mg bid for 7 days
Naproxen + prochlorperazine	550 mg + 10 mg over 3–7 days	550 mg + 10 mg bid for 7 days
Other		
Tizanidine	2–4 mg tid	2 mg bid and 4mg hs × 10 days
Olanzapine	2.5–10 mg bid	2.5–10 mg qhs × 5 days
Methylergonovine	0.2 mg	1po tid × 14 days

Peripheral procedures

Peripheral anesthetic procedures, such as nerve blocks, offer the potential for rapid headache relief with minimal AEs. Greater occipital nerve blocks have been used for migraine and reports are generally positive, especially for patients with allodynia. We use local anesthetics such as lidocaine (1% or 2% solution), longer-acting bupivacaine (0.25%–0.5%) solution, or a combination of two agents, for the blocks. Corticosteroids are sometimes added, but these drugs have no proven additional benefit, except in cluster headache (Figure 5.1, Table 5.17).

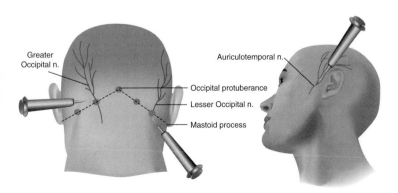

FIGURE 5.1 Nerve block procedures in migraine.

TABLE 5.17 Nerve Block Procedures in Migraine

Nerve Block Site	Location
Greater occipital	Medial to occipital artery, 1/3 of the distance between occipital protuberance and mastoid process
Lesser occipital	Lateral to occipital artery, 2/3 of the distance between occipital protuberance and mastoid process
Auriculotemporal	Anterior to the ear, superior to the posterior portion of the zygoma
Supratrochlear[a]	Above the medial border of the eyebrow
Supraorbital[a]	Above the eyebrow, about 2 cm lateral to supratrochlear nerve

[a] One can palpate the supraorbital notch easily and inject immediately above it in the eyebrow.

Muscle spasm is common in migraine, and focal trigger point injections into the muscle provide many patients immediate relief. Unlike nerve blocks, trigger point injection focuses on reducing palpable spasm and may not produce anesthesia. Common sites of trigger point injections include the paraspinal, splenius capitus, trapezius, and masseter muscles.

Future Directions

Although many treatment options are available, some migraine sufferers still experience profound disability. Advances in our understanding of migraine pathophysiology are leading to new treatments. Calcitonin gene-related peptide (CGRP) is important in migraine, and CGRP antagonists, which are effective and well tolerated, will soon become available. Other potential targets include adenosine receptor agonists, glutamate receptor antagonists, and nitric oxide synthase inhibitors. Carbon dioxide NS appears promising based on early clinical observations, and there may even be a role for nonmedication alternatives, such as repetitive transcranial magnetic stimulation for acute migraine with aura.

REFERENCES

Chou R, Fanciullo GJ, Fine PG, et al. Clinical guidelines for the use of chronic opioid therapy in chronic noncancer pain. *J Pain.* 2009;10(2):113–130.e22.

Evans RW, Young WB. Droperidol and other neuroleptics/antiemetics for the management of migraine. *Headache.* 2003;43(7):811–813.

Ferrari MD, Roon KI, Lipton RB, Goadsby PJ. Oral triptans (serotonin 5-HT(1B/1D) agonists) in acute migraine treatment: a meta-analysis of 53 trials. *Lancet.* 2001;358(9294):1668–1675.

Gillman PK. Triptans, serotonin agonists, and serotonin syndrome (serotonin toxicity): a review. *Headache*. 2010;50(2):264.

Saper JR, Lake AE III. Continuous opioid therapy (COT) is rarely advisable for refractory chronic daily headache: limited efficacy, risks, and proposed guidelines. *Headache.* 2008;48(6):838–849.

6 Migraine: Preventing Attacks

INTRODUCTION

Preventive treatment is one of the most important aspects of migraine management. This does not always involve medication, and in fact, it does not always revolve around ingesting therapeutic substances. Behavioral treatments and lifestyle modifications are often just as effective and are always advisable in adjunctive management of migraine (Chapter 11). This chapter will focus on medications effective in preventing recurrent migraine attacks and how to use them. First, let us review why and when to institute preventive measures.

MIGRAINE PREVENTION: WHY?

Migraine is a disabling disorder that detracts from the joy of life. Yet, migraine affects the patient not only during attacks but also between attacks. Interictal phenomena of hypersensitivity to certain stimuli are well-documented, and some patients find this quite bothersome. Migraines are often triggered by everyday occurrences and exposures, requiring patients to limit their activities, avoid certain foods, and even forego their career pursuits. Many patients find themselves refraining from social events for fear of a migraine attack.

Migraine is a costly condition. Triptans are expensive (as much as $50 per dose) and do not always work, requiring more adjunctive medications, or even worse, visits to the emergency department for intensive evaluation and treatment. Reduced productivity and missed days from work also result from migraine. Some patients cannot work at all and must rely on disability income or be dependent upon another individual to survive. Taking direct and indirect expenditures into account, the estimated annual cost of migraine in the United States is over $20 billion.

Finally, migraine affects not only the patient but also the patient's family. A parent sick with a migraine cannot care for his/her children and must rely on a spouse or someone else; and this may require that the helper take time off work or miss other planned activities. Friends live with the uncertainty of whether a person with migraine will be able to fulfill social commitments, and they may find themselves worrying about the patient's well being. Loved ones do not wish to see the patient suffer. It can be especially hard on young children, who commonly harbor fears that their parent is gravely ill. Prevention can address all of the aforementioned concerns (Table 6.1).

TABLE 6.1 Goals of Preventive Treatment

- Reduce attack frequency, intensity, and duration
- Improve responsiveness to acute medication
- Improve function and reduce disability
- Reduce costs
- Prevent disease progression

MIGRAINE PREVENTION: WHEN?

Prevention is necessary when migraine causes undue distress, dysfunction, and spending of healthcare dollars (Table 6.2).

The recommendation to start preventive treatment when headaches occur more than once weekly is supported by data from a large population of episodic migraine patients (Figure 6.1).

TABLE 6.2 When to Consider Prevention

- Migraine significantly interferes with the patient's daily routine, despite acute treatment
- Frequent attacks (>1/week) with risk of chronic daily headache or medication overuse headache
- Acute medications ineffective, contraindicated, overused, or cause troublesome AEs
- Patient preference
- Presence of uncommon migraine conditions with potentially disastrous consequences
  - Hemiplegic migraine
  - Basilar migraine
  - Migraine with prolonged aura
  - Migrainous infarction
- Treating attacks is excessively costly (expensive acute medications, frequent visits to office or ER, frequent use of diagnostic testing when attacks mimic secondary headache disorder, e.g., hemiplegic migraine)

Abbreviations: AEs, adverse events; ER, emergency room.

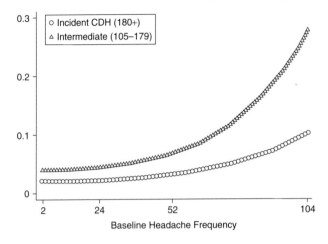

FIGURE 6.1 Headache frequency at baseline predicts progression to chronic daily headache at 1 year. The top line shows the predicted incidence of intermediate frequent headaches (105–179 headache days/year) and the bottom line shows the predicted incidence of chronic daily headache (180+ headache days/year). The inflection point for progression occurs a little beyond 52 headache days per year (or average of once weekly).
Source: Scher AI, et al. *Pain*. 2003;106(1–2):81–89.

MIGRAINE PREVENTION: HOW?

When deciding to start preventive therapy, there are many medications to choose from. The ideal medication is highly effective across a broad population, has few side effects (or advantageous ones), and does not interfere with (or even better, enhances) the treatment of coexistent conditions. Once the treatment is selected, set realistic expectations. Inform the patient of common and uncommon side effects and how to manage them. Explain that preventive treatment takes time to work (several weeks if not months) and is unlikely to eliminate attacks entirely, but will make them far more manageable in terms of reduced frequency, intensity, and duration, and should improve responsiveness to acute treatment. Acute medication overuse may interfere with the effectiveness of preventive medications, and steps must be taken to reduce acute medication use (e.g., behavioral measures). Start with 10% to 30% of the target preventive medication dose and increase incrementally and gradually (5–14 days between dose escalations). If the first preventive trial fails, try something from another therapeutic class, and revisit any issue of medication overuse. If multiple single trials fail, consider using two or more preventive medications in combination. When results seem suboptimal, daily calendars can be useful in establishing whether any type of gains are being made (frequency, intensity, responsiveness to acute treatment) and can also reveal unrecognized medication overuse. For women of childbearing potential, ensure contraception is adequate. Finally, ongoing assessment of the success and appropriateness of preventive treatment is essential. Have patients keep track of their headaches to monitor for changes in frequency, intensity, responsiveness to acute medications, and temporal pattern. Sometimes these changes are not obvious and require a headache calendar to document them. Many patients are mistaken about their baseline headache frequency and patterns. Once adequate control has been attained and maintained for 6 months, consider tapering preventive medication. Patients can often taper medication without worsening and can maintain control with lifestyle changes and nonprescription supplements (Table 6.3). A recent placebo-controlled, double-blind study has shown that the effects of 6 months of preventive treatment with topiramate (Topamax) can last for at least 6 months after discontinuation.

How do preventive medications work? Many believe that preventive medications reduce neuronal hyperexcitability. Evidence from an animal model of migraine supports this: preventives raise the threshold for cortical spreading depression. Endothelial stabilization may be another mechanism, because angiotensin converting enzyme inhibitors, as well as angiotensin receptor blockers, have demonstrated preventive benefit. As more treatments are discovered to be helpful in migraine prevention (indeed, most are serendipitous and not engineered), more light will be shed on the pathophysiological underpinnings of the disorder.

TABLE 6.3 Principles of Preventive Treatment

1. Choose based on efficacy, AE profile, coexistent conditions, and diagnosis
2. Communicate realistic expectations
3. Start at low dose and gradually increase until efficacy achieved, side effects develop, or ceiling dose reached
4. Benefit develops slowly (months); often not fully effective until overuse eliminated
5. If first choice fails, choose second from another therapeutic class
6. Monotherapy preferred, but combination therapy often necessary
7. Avoid pregnancy
8. Evaluate therapy
   - Use calendar
   - Slowly taper to lowest effective dose (and stop) if headaches well controlled

Abbreviation: AE, adverse event.

MIGRAINE PREVENTION: WHAT?

Preventive medications generally come in four categories: anticonvulsants, antidepressants, antihypertensives, and others. The following tables detail examples from each category, relative efficacies, starting and target doses, and considerations for coexistent/comorbid conditions. It is also important to remember, especially in patients with comorbidities, that vigilance must be maintained to avoid unnecessary polypharmacy and drug-drug interactions (Tables 6.4–6.7).

TABLE 6.4 Some Useful Preventive Medications

Anticonvulsants
    Divalproex[a]
    Gabapentin
    Topiramate[a]
Antidepressants
    TCAs (nortriptyline, amitriptyline, protriptyline)
    SSRIs/SNRIs (fluoxetine, venlafaxine, duloxetine)
β-Blockers
    Propranolol[a]
    Timolol[a]
    Atenolol
    Metoprolol
Calcium channel blockers
    Verapamil
    Diltiazem
Angiotensin system
    ACE inhibitors (lisinopril)
    Receptor antagonists (candesartan, olmesartan, irbesartan)
Others
    5-HT antagonists (methysergide[b], methergine)
    "Natural" remedies (riboflavin, coenzyme Q10, magnesium, petasites)
    Onabotulinum neurotoxin[c]
    Minocycline
    Memantine
    Atypical neuroleptics

Abbreviations: ACE, angiotensin-converting enzyme; TCAs, tricyclic antidepressants.
[a] FDA approved for the prevention of episodic migraine.
[b] Not available in US.
[c] FDA approved for the prevention of chronic migraine.

TABLE 6.5 US Consortium Recommendations

Group 1	Group 2	Group 3	Group 4	Group 5
Anticonvulsants	***Anticonvulsants***	***Anticonvulsants***	***Anticonvulsants***	***Anticonvulsants***
Topiramate	Gabapentin	Carbamazepine	Tiagabine	Lamotrigine
Divalproex sodium				Oxcarbazepine
	Antidepressants	***Calcium channel blockers***	***Antidepressants***	Clonazepam
Antidepressants	Fluoxetine	Verapamil	Nortriptyline	
Amitriptyline	Venlafaxine	Diltiazem	Protriptyline	***Others***
		Nimodipine	Imipramine	Acetazolamide
β-Blockers	***β-Blockers***	Nifedipine	Doxepin	Lanepitant
Timolol	Atenolol	Nicardipine	Fluvoxamine	Montelukast
Propranolol	Nadolol		Paroxetine	Omega-3
Metoprolol		***α-Agonists***	Sertraline	Vitamin E
	Angiotensin system	Clonidine[a]	Phenelzine	
Serotonin Antagonist	Lisinopril	Guanfacine		
Methysergide	Candesartan		***β-Blockers***	
			Pindolol	
Serotonin Agonist	***Other***		Acebutolol	
Frovatriptan[a]	Coenzyme Q 10		Bisoprolol	
	Riboflavin			

Other
Petasides (butterbur)

Feverfew

Serotonin agonist
Naratriptan[a]
Zolmitriptan[a]

NSAIDs
Aspirin
Fenoprofen
Flurbiprofen
Ibuprofen
Ketoprofen
Mefenamic acid[a]
Naproxen (sodium)

Serotonin antagonist
Methylergonovine

Anticoagulants
Coumadin
Acenocoumarol
Picotamide

Abbreviation: NSAIDs, nonsteroidal anti-inflammatory drugs.

Groups of medications used for migraine prevention based on levels of evidence for efficacy according to the Quality Standards Subcommittee of the American Academy of Neurology

[a] For short-term prophylaxis of menstrually related migraine

- Group 1: medications with proven high efficacy based on at least two Class-I trials (should be used).
- Group 2: medications probably effective based on one Class-I or at least two Class-II trials (should be considered).
- Group 3: medications possibly effective based on one Class-II trial or at least two Class-III trials, or conflicting studies (may be considered).
- Group 4: medications cannot be recommended based on inadequate or conflicting data (Class-IV trials or no trials) (we cannot recommend these drugs one way or the other but some are used frequently—for example, nortriptyline).
- Group 5: medications probably ineffective (based on one Class-I or at least two Class-II trials (should not be considered).

TABLE 6.6 Using Various Preventive Medications

Drug	Starting Dose	Target Dose	Side Effects	Monitoring/Comments
Anticonvulsants (Although used as mood stabilizers, be vigilant for destabilization of mood with any of these.)				
Topiramate	25 mg	100–200 mg/day	Sedation, incoordination cognitive impairment, paresthesias, weight loss, hair loss, calcium phosphate kidney stones	If patient develops kidney stone, make sure it is analyzed
Divalproex sodium	250 mg	1500–2000 mg/day	Nausea, weight gain, polycystic ovaries	Monitor CBC, hepatic function, and drug level; many drug-drug interactions
Gabapentin	300 mg	3600–4800 mg/day	Weight gain	Pharmacologically "clean"
Zonisamide	25 mg	150–300 mg/day	Similar to topiramate, but usually less intense	
Levetiracetam	250 mg	2000–3000 mg/day	Violent behavior (rare)	Usually not useful, negative trial published, but has helped some patients
Lamotrigine	25 mg	100–200 mg/day	Stevens-Johnson syndrome occurs if dose escalated too quickly	Usually not useful, except with prominent aura
Antidepressants (All of the following can cause sexual dysfunction; caution with bipolar patients, adolescents, and older patients because of potential for mood destabilization and suicidality.)				
Tricyclics			Sedation, dry mouth, constipation, weight gain	
Amitriptyline	10 mg	30–50 mg		Monitor levels and EKG
				Metabolized to nortriptyline

Drug	Starting dose	Target dose	Side effects	Comments
Nortriptyline	10 mg	30–50 mg		Less sedation (can be energizing) and less weight gain, but more dryness
Protriptyline	5 mg tid	10–20 mg tid		
Imipramine	10 mg	30–50 mg		
Doxepin	10 mg	30–50 mg		
Tetracyclic				
Mirtazapine	7.5 mg	15–30 mg	Sedation, weight gain	Taper slowly, withdrawal can be very uncomfortable.
SNRIs				
Venlafaxine	25–37.5 mg	150–300 mg/day	Nausea, palpitations, weight gain	Perhaps most useful for patients with anxiety or fibromyalgia
Duloxetine	20–30 mg	60–120 mg/day		
SSRIs				
Fluoxetine	10 mg	40 mg/day		May only benefit the anxious patient
Sertraline	25–50 mg	100–200 mg/day		
MAOIs			Hypotension, weight gain	Many dangerous drug-drug interactions, low tyramine diet required, not good for unreliable/noncompliant patients
Phenelzine	15 mg bid/tid	90 mg/day		Can escalate rapidly as tolerated
Tranylcypromine	10 mg bid/tid	60 mg/day		Increase q 1–3 weeks

Continued

TABLE 6.6 Using Various Preventive Medications (*Continued*)

Drug	Starting Dose	Target Dose	Side Effects	Monitoring/Comments
Selegeline transdermal	6 mg/day	12 mg/day		Increase q 2 weeks, no dietary restrictions at 6 mg/day dose
Isocarboxazid	10 mg bid	60 mg/day		
Antihypertensives (All of the following can cause hypotension, fatigue; can be used in patients with normal or low blood pressure; just start low and go slow.)				
β-Blockers			Depression, bronchospasm	
Propranolol	10–60 mg	120 mg		
Timolol	2.5–10 mg/day	20 mg/day		
Metoprolol	25 mg	50–100 mg/day		
Atenolol	25 mg	50–100 mg/day		
Nadolol				
Calcium channel blockers				
Verapamil	40–120 mg/day	240–720 mg/day	Constipation, peripheral edema, PR prolongation	EKG at baseline, with dose escalations, and at least twice yearly thereafter
Diltiazem	30–120 mg/day	360–540 mg/day	Constipation, peripheral edema, PR prolongation	EKG at baseline, with dose escalations, and at least twice yearly thereafter
Flunarizine	5 mg	10 mg	Weight gain	Not available in United States
Nifedipine	10–30 mg/day	60–180 mg/day	Constipation, peripheral edema, arrhythmia	
Nimodipine	30–120 mg/day	120–240 mg day	Edema, arrhythmia	Very expensive, monitor hepatic enzymes

Angiotensin system				
Lisinopril	2.5–5 mg	10–20 mg		
Candesartan	4–8 mg	16 mg		
Irbesartan	75 mg	150–300 mg		
Olmesartan	5 mg	20–40 mg	Cough	
Others				
Methysergide	2 mg bid	2 mg tid/qid	Nausea	Not available in United States, 4-week drug holiday or CT of chest/abdomen/pelvis every 6 months, not for use in patients with vascular risks
Methergine	0.2 mg bid/tid	0.4 mg tid	Nausea	4-week drug holiday or CT of chest/abdomen/pelvis every 6 months, not for use in patients with vascular risks
Onabotulinum neurotoxin	100 units	300 units		
Cyproheptadine	2–4 mg	4–12 mg	Sedation, weight gain, antihistamine effects	
Memantine	5 mg	20–40 mg/day	Insomnia, tension-type headache	
Minocycline	50–100 mg	100–200 mg/day	Nausea	

Continued

TABLE 6.6 Using Various Preventive Medications (*Continued*)

Drug	Starting Dose	Target Dose	Side Effects	Monitoring/Comments
Natural remedies				
Petasides	150 mg/day	150 mg/day	Burping	Dose may be reduced to 100 mg/day once efficacy established, can be expensive and hard to find, Petadolex brand recommended because of regulated manufacturing
Riboflavin	200–400 mg/day	200–400 mg/day	Bright yellow urine	
Magnesium	200 mg/day	1200 mg/day	Diarrhea	High doses not always necessary for benefit
Coenzyme Q 10	150–300 mg/day	300 mg/day and up		Energizing, antioxidant properties, safe to take high doses if added benefit demonstrated, expensive

Abbreviations: CBC, complete blood count; MAOIs, monoamine oxidase inhibitors; SNRIs, serotonin–norepinephrine reuptake inhibitors; SSRIs, selective serotonin reuptake inhibitors.

TABLE 6.7 Considering Comorbidities

Drug	Efficacy	Side Effects	Relative Indications	Relative Contraindications
Anticonvulsants				
Topiramate	4+	2+	Epilepsy, obesity, MOH?	Calcium phosphate kidney stones
Divalproex	4+	2+	Epilepsy, bipolar disorder	Obesity, hepatic dysfunction, bleeding disorder, fertile woman
Gabapentin	2+	2+	Epilepsy, neuropathic pain	Obesity
Antidepressants				
TCAs	4+	2+	Depression, anxiety, insomnia, other pain disorder	Bipolar disorder, heart block, urinary retention, obesity
SSRIs	2+	1+	Depression, anxiety, OCD	Bipolar disorder
SNRIs	2+	2+	Depression, anxiety, fibromyalgia	Bipolar disorder, hypertension
Antihypertensives				
β-Blockers	4+	2+	Hypertension, angina	Asthma, depression, congestive heart failure, diabetes, Raynaud's disease
Calcium channel blockers	2+	1+	Raynaud's disease, migraine with unusual aura	Heart block, chronic constipation
ACE-I	2+	1+	Hypertension	Chronic cough
ARB	2+	1+	Hypertension	Chronic cough
Others				
Riboflavin	2+	1+	Preference for nutraceutical	None
Coenzyme Q 10	2+	1+	Fatigue	None
Magnesium	1+	1+	Constipation	Diarrhea, renal impairment
Petasides	2+	1+	Preference for nutraceutical	None
Onabotulinum neurotoxin	2+	1+	Chronic migraine	Local infection, neuromuscular disorder

ACE-I, angiotensin-converting enzyme inhibitor; ARB, angiotensin receptor blocker; MOH, medication overuse headache; SNRIs, serotonin-norepinephrine reuptake inhibitors; SSRIs, selective serotonin reuptake inhibitors; TCAs, tricyclic antidepressants.

REFERENCES

Ayata C, Jin H, Kudo C, Dalkara T, Moskowitz MA. Suppression of cortical spreading depression in migraine prophylaxis. *Annals of Neurology.* 2006;59(4),652–661.

Diener HC, Agosti R, Allais G, et al. Cessation versus continuation of 6-month migraine preventive therapy with topiramate (PROMPT): a randomized, double-blind, placebo-controlled trial. *Lancet Neurology.* 2007;6(12),1054–1062.

Dodick DW, Silberstein SD. Migraine prevention. *Practical Neurology.* 2007;7(6),383–393.

Munakata J, Hazard E, Serrano D, et al. Economic burden of transformed migraine: results from the American migraine prevalence and prevention (AMPP) study. *Headache.* 2009;49(4),498–508.

Scher AI, Stewart WF, Ricci JA, Lipton RB. Factors associated with the onset and remission of chronic daily headache in a population-based study. *Pain.* 2003;106(1–2),81–89.

7 Hormones and Headache

There is a link between migraine and the female sex hormones—estrogen and progesterone. Migraine occurs more frequently in adult women (18%) than in men (6%), although prevalence is equal in children. Migraine develops most frequently in the second decade, with the peak incidence occurring with adolescence. Many migrainous women experience menstrual migraine (MM) mainly at the time of menses (menstrually related migraine [MRM]) and some experience it exclusively with menses (pure menstrual migraine [PMM]). Migraine may worsen during the first trimester of pregnancy and although many women become headache-free during the last two trimesters, 25% have no change in their migraine. MM typically improves with pregnancy, perhaps due to sustained high estrogen levels. Hormonal replacement with estrogens can exacerbate migraine, and oral contraceptives (OCs) can change its character and frequency. Migraine prevalence decreases with advancing age (>50) but may regress or worsen at menopause. Changes in the headache pattern with OC use and during menarche, menstruation, pregnancy, or menopause are related to changes in estrogen levels (Table 7.1).

TABLE 7.1 Sex Hormone Milestones

- Menarche
- Menstruation
- Hormonal contraception
- Pregnancy
- Menopause
- Hormonal replacement

MENSTRUAL MIGRAINE

Migraine can occur before or during menstruation. When migraine occurs before menstruation, features of premenstrual syndrome (PMS) may also be present. MM is not typically associated with aura (Table 7.2).

MM is defined (ICHD-2) as attacks that occur during a 5-day interval that extends from 2 days before through 3 days after the onset of menses in at least two out of three menstrual cycles (Table 7.3).

TABLE 7.2 Types of Menstrual Migraine

MRM
    Attacks occur days −2 to +3 of menses and at other times
PMM
    Attacks only occur days −2 to +3 of menses
Premenstrual migraine
    Attacks occur days −7 to −2 before menses

Abbreviations: MRM, menstrually related migraine; PMM, pure menstrual migraine.

TABLE 7.3 Menstrual Migraine: Diagnostic Criteria

PMM without aura
    Diagnostic criteria
    A. Attacks, in a menstruating woman, fulfilling criteria for 1.1 *Migraine without aura*
    B. Attacks occur exclusively on day 1 ± 2 (i.e., days −2 to +3) of menstruation in at least two out of three menstrual cycles and at no other times of the cycle
The first day of menstruation is day 1 and the preceding day is day −1; there is no day 0.
MRM without aura
    Diagnostic criteria
    A. Attacks, in a menstruating woman, fulfilling criteria for 1.1 *Migraine without aura*
    B. Attacks occur on day 1 ± 2 (i.e., days −2 to +3) of menstruation in at least two out of three menstrual cycles and additionally at other times of the cycle

Abbreviations: MRM, menstrually related migraine; PMM, pure menstrual migraine.

Treatment Overview

There are two pharmacologic approaches to treatment: acute and preventive. Women who have migraine predominantly with their menses can simply be treated perimenstrually with short-term miniprophylaxis.

Acute treatment

Drugs commonly used for the acute treatment of MM include nonsteroidal anti-inflammatory drugs (NSAIDs); the combination of aspirin, acetaminophen, and caffeine; dihydroergotamine (DHE); and the triptans. All the triptans are effective in subcutaneous, oral, and intranasal formulations. All are as effective for MRM as for non-MRM.

    If severe MRM cannot be controlled with NSAIDs, DHE, triptans, analgesics, opioids, corticosteroids, or neuroleptics (chlorpromazine, haloperidol,

TABLE 7.4 Preventive Treatment Strategies for MM

1. Perimenstrual use of standard preventive drugs
2. Perimenstrual use of nonstandard preventive drugs
   - NSAIDs
   - Ergotamine and its derivatives
   - Triptans
   - Magnesium
3. Hormonal therapy
   - Estrogens (with or without androgens or progestin)
   - COCs
   - Synthetic androgens (Danazol)
   - Antiestrogen (Tamoxifen)
   - Medical oophorectomy (GnRH analogues)
4. Dopamine agonists (Bromocriptine)

Abbreviations: COCs, combined oral contraceptives; GnRH, gonadotropin-releasing hormone; MM, menstrual migraine; NSAIDs, nonsteroidal anti-inflammatory drugs.

thiothixene, droperidol), a course of intravenous (IV) DHE can be tried. Women with frequent, severe MRM are candidates for preventive therapy.

Women who are already using preventive medication and continue to have MRM can increase the dose prior to their menses (Table 7.4).

Women can also be treated perimenstrually with short-term prophylaxis (Table 7.5). NSAIDs in adequate doses can be used preventively 1 to 2 days before the expected onset of headache and continued for the duration of vulnerability.

DHE can be used preventively at the time of menses without significant risk of developing ergot dependence. Oral sumatriptan (25 mg tid), naratriptan (1 mg bid), and zolmitriptan given 2 to 3 days before the expected headache onset and continued for a total of 5 days are probably effective. Frovatriptan (a loading dose of 5 mg followed by 2.5 mg bid) was more effective than placebo when used for short-term prevention of MRM.

TABLE 7.5 Short-term Prevention in MM

Drug	Dosing	Dose (mg po)
NSAIDs		
Naproxen	tid	275–500
Ketoprofen	bid	75–150
Ibuprofen	bid	200–400
Triptans		
Sumatriptan	tid	25
Naratriptan	bid	1
Zolmitriptan	bid	5
Frovatriptan	bid	2.5 (loading dose 5)

Abbreviation: NSAIDs, nonsteroidal anti-inflammatory drugs.

If severe MRM cannot be controlled by standard acute and preventive treatment, hormonal therapy may be indicated (Table 7.6). Successful hormonal therapy of MRM has been reported with estrogens (alone or combined with progesterone or testosterone), combined OCs (COCs), synthetic androgens, estrogen modulators and antagonists, and medical oophorectomy with gonadotropin-releasing hormone (GnRH) analog with or without add-back therapy and prolactin release inhibitors. Progesterone is not effective in the treatment of headache or the symptoms of PMS, despite many favorable anecdotal reports.

The estradiol cutaneous patch provides a relatively stable plasma-estrogen level over the time of application. A serum estradiol level of at least 60 to 80 pg/mL is required (a TTS patch >50) to prevent estrogen-withdrawal migraine.

Combinations of estrogens and progestogens, or progestogens alone in the form of OCs, can be used (see OC section). Women can extend the active OCs

TABLE 7.6 Hormonal Manipulation

Estrogens (with or without progesterone)

Estradiol

■ Cream: cyclic

■ Cutaneous patch: cyclic or continuous

OCs

■ Cyclic OC: some women's migraine will occur only menstrually and with less severity

■ Continuous OCs
  • 3 months without placebo (Seasonale, Seasonique)
  • New formulation (Lybrel) designed for continuous use

Transdermal estrogens

■ Use patch perimenstrually
  • TTS 25, 50, 100

■ Need serum estradiol level >60 pg/mL to be effective
  • Requires strength >TTS 50

SERMs

■ Raloxifen: estrogen antagonist on uterus and breast. Estrogen agonist on bone and serum lipids

Others

■ Neither hysterectomy nor oophorectomy is effective in the treatment of migraine

■ GnRH agonist administration, alone or with add-back therapy, may be effective for carefully selected patients who have severe, perimenstrual migraine headaches, although results are modest

Abbreviations: OCs, oral contraceptives; GnRH, gonadotropin-releasing hormone; SERMs, selective estrogen receptor modulators.

for 6 to 12 weeks. New commercial preparations (Seasonale and Seasonique) that allow for four menstrual cycles per year are now available, whereas a new formulation (Lybrel) is designed for continuous use. Compared with the standard 21/7-day OC regimen, a 168-day extended placebo-free regimen led to a decrease in headache severity along with improvement in work productivity and involvement in activities (Table 7.6).

MIGRAINE, CONTRACEPTIVES, AND ISCHEMIC STROKE

Hormonal contraceptive steroids are available as OCs, transdermal combination patches, subcutaneous implants, depo injections, and vaginal rings (Table 7.7). By eliminating most, if not all, pill-free intervals, long-cycle

TABLE 7.7 Oral Contraceptives

Type	Progestin (mg)/Ethinyl Estradiol (mcg)
Combination Monophasic	
Second generation	
Ethynodiol diacetate	1/30,1/35,1/50
Levonorgestrel[a]	0.1/20, 0.15/30
Norethindrone	0.4/35, 0.5/35, 1/20, 1/35, 1/50, 1.5/30, 1/50[b]
Norethindrone acetate	0.05/35, 0.1/20, 0.1/35, 0.15/30
Norgestrel	0.3/30, 0.5/50
Third generation	
Desogestrel	0.15/30
Norgestimate	0.25/35
Drospirenone	3.0/20, 3.0/30
Biphasic	
Norethindrone	0.5/35 and 1/35
Desogestrel	0.15/20, placebo, and 0.15/10; 0.15/20, placebo, and 0.0/10
Triphasic	
Norethindrone	1/20, 1/30, 1/35; 0.5/35, 0.75/35, 1/35; 0.5/35, 1/35, 0.5/35
Levonorgestrel	0.05/30, 0.075/40, 0.125/30
Norgestimate	0.18/35, 0.215/35, 0.25/35
Progestin only	
Ethynodiol diacetate	0.5
Levonorgestrel	0.030
Norethindrone	0.35
Norgestrel	0.075

[a] Available as 84 active tablets and 7 placebo tablets (Seasonale).

[b] Mestranol.

regimens with infrequent bleeds are a variable option. Absolute contraindications to OC use include a history of ischemic stroke; vascular disease, including thromboembolism, thrombophlebitis, and atherosclerosis; and systemic disease that can affect the vascular system, such as lupus erythematosus or diabetes with retinopathy or nephropathy. Other contraindications to OC use include uncontrolled hypertension and cigarette smoking by women older than 35 years. Women who are given OCs must be followed for headache aggravation or the development of neurologic symptoms.

OC use is relatively safe for women younger than age 35 who have migraine without aura. Women with intractable MM or a history of headache relief with OCs are particularly good candidates for a trial of OCs. Women younger than age 35 who have migraine with typical aura can probably safely use OCs, but they should be used with caution.

Guidelines from the World Health Organization, the American College of Obstetrics and Gynecology, and the International Headache Society discourage the use of estrogen-containing contraceptives by women who have migraine with aura and urge caution for those who have migraine without aura and are older than 35 years or have other risk factors for thromboembolic complications, such as smoking, obesity, or hypertension.

MENOPAUSE

Menopause is the permanent cessation of menstruation. The average age of menopause is between 51 and 52 years, with a range of 40 to 60 years. Menopause is associated with both early and late symptoms. Many women go through the menopausal transition with few or no symptoms, whereas some have significant or even disabling symptoms. Although migraine prevalence decreases with advancing age, migraine can either regress or worsen at menopause. Migraine may increase in frequency and severity in the perimenopausal periods, probably because of erratic estrogen secretion at these times. Most women experience migraine improvement after physiologic menopause. In one study, two thirds of women with prior migraine improved with physiologic menopause; in contrast, two thirds of women who had surgical menopause had a worsening of migraine (Table 7.8).

Hormone Replacement Therapy and Headaches

Hormone replacement therapy (HRT) can be with estrogen alone (estrogen replacement therapy [ERT]) or combined with a progestin. Oral, but not transdermal, HRT is often associated with worsening of migraine. Headaches that develop as a result of HRT may be difficult to manage. Several empirical strategies are useful (Table 7.9).

TABLE 7.8 Menopausal Symptoms

Early
  Hot flushes
  ■ Associated with pulses of
    hypothalamic activity that
    lead to pulses of luteinizing hormone
  ■ Atrophic vaginitis
  Psychologic and somatic complaints
  ■ Depression
  ■ Anxiety
  ■ Fatigue
  ■ Dizziness
  ■ Insomnia
  ■ Altered libido
  ■ Loss of concentration
  ■ Headache
Late
  ■ Dyspareunia
  ■ Hirsutism
  ■ Reduced breast size
  ■ Dry skin
  ■ Osteoporosis
  ■ Arteriosclerotic
    cardiovascular disease

TABLE 7.9 HRT and Migraine

Estrogens
  1. Reduce estrogen dose
  2. Change estrogen type from conjugated estrogen to pure estradiol to
     synthetic estrogen to pure estrone
  3. Convert from interrupted to continuous dosing
  4. Convert from oral to parenteral dosing
  5. Add androgens
  6. Switch to selective estrogen receptor modulator
Progestin
  1. Switch from interrupted (cyclic) to continuous lower dose
  2. Change progestin type
  3. Change delivery system (oral to vaginal)
  4. Discontinue progestin (periodic endometrial biopsy or vaginal ultrasound)

Reducing the dose of estrogen or changing the estrogen type from conjugated estrogen to pure estradiol, ethinyl estradiol, or estrone may reduce headache. Changing from interrupted to continuous administration may be very effective if the headaches are associated with estrogen withdrawal. Techniques may be combined. The estradiol cutaneous patch, which provides a physiologic ratio of estradiol to estrone and a steady-state concentration of estrogen, has been associated with fewer headache side effects. The new selective estrogen receptor modulator (SERM), raloxifene, can be used if a woman requires, but cannot tolerate, estrogen.

Progestins, used to prevent endometrial hyperplasia, can cause headache, particularly if used cyclically. Giving a lower dose of a progestin continuously can often control this effect. Another strategy is to change the type of progestin used. One can use targeted drug delivery, like the progesterone-containing vaginal gel. This maximizes progesterone's effect on the uterus while minimizing its potential adverse effects, including headaches. Progestogens, particularly norethisterone and megestrol, can relieve or reduce hot flushes independently of estrogen.

MIGRAINE AND PREGNANCY

Most women with migraine improve during pregnancy—women without aura more commonly than women with aura. Some women have their first attack during pregnancy. Migraine often recurs postpartum and can begin for the first time in general.

The Food and Drug Administration (FDA) lists five categories of labeling for drug use in pregnancy.

Category A: Controlled human studies show no risk.
Category B: No evidence of risk in humans, but no controlled human studies.
Category C: Risk to humans has not been ruled out.
Category D: Positive evidence of risk from human and/or animal studies.
Category X: Contraindicated in pregnancy.

An alternate rating system is TERIS, an automated teratogen information resource wherein the rating for each drug or agent is based on a consensus of expert opinion and the literature (Table 7.10).

The major concerns in managing the pregnant patient are the effects of both the medication and the disease on the fetus. Medication use should be limited;

TABLE 7.10 TERIS Compared to FDA Labeling

N	None (A)
N-Min	None-minimal (A)
Min	Minimal (B)
Min-S	Minimal-small (D)
S	Small
S-Mod	Small-Moderate
Mod	Moderate
H	High (X)
U	Undetermined (C)
Unl	Unlikely

Equivalent FDA ratings in parenthesis.

however, it is not contraindicated during pregnancy. Many women can manage their headaches with reassurance and nonpharmacologic means of coping, such as ice, massage, and biofeedback. Some women, however, will continue to have severe, intractable headaches, sometimes associated with nausea, vomiting, and possible dehydration.

Acute Treatment

Individual attacks should be treated with rest, reassurance, and ice packs. For headaches that do not respond to nonpharmacologic treatment, symptomatic drugs are indicated. NSAIDs, acetaminophen (alone or with codeine), codeine alone, or other opioids can be used during pregnancy. However, all opioids can produce maternal and neonatal addiction. Their use for prolonged periods of time and in high doses at term is contraindicated (Tables 7.11 and 7.12).

Mild nausea can be treated with phosphorylated carbohydrate solution (emetrol: an oral solution containing balanced amounts of fructose and glucose with orthophosphoric acid) or doxylamine succinate and vitamin B6 (pyridoxine). More severe nausea may require injections or suppositories. Trimethobenzamide, chlorpromazine, prochlorperazine, and promethazine can all be used. They are available orally, parenterally, and in suppository form. We frequently use promethazine and prochlorperazine suppositories.

TABLE 7.11 Acute Treatment

■ Aspirin in low intermittent doses does not have a significant teratogenic risk, although large doses, especially if given near term, may be associated with maternal and fetal bleeding	if possible, and certainly during the last trimester
■ NSAIDs may be safely taken for pain during the first trimester of pregnancy. However, their use should be limited during later pregnancy, as some NSAIDs may constrict or close the fetal ductus arteriosus	• Barbiturate and benzodiazepine use should be limited • Ergotamine and DHE should be avoided
■ The most potent inhibitors of prostaglandin synthesis, such as salicylates and indomethacin, should probably be avoided throughout pregnancy	• All triptans are rated as FDA pregnancy class C, which means that "safety in human pregnancy has not been determined" and that "potential benefits should justify potential risks" if the decision to use the drug during pregnancy is made. Triptans should probably be avoided, but this belief is controversial

Abbreviations: DHE, dihydroergotamine; NSAIDs, nonsteroidal anti-inflammatory drugs.

TABLE 7.12 Ergots and Triptans

	Fetal Risk	
	FDA	TERIS
Ergots		
DHE	X	Min
Ergotamine	X	U
Triptans		
Almotriptan	C	U
Eletriptan	C	U
Frovatriptan	C	U
Naratriptan	C	U
Rizatriptan	C	U
Sumatriptan	C	U
Zolmitriptan	C	Unl

Abbreviation: DHE, dihydroergotamine.

Corticosteroids can be used occasionally (some suggest limiting its use during the first trimester). Some use prednisone in preference to dexamethasone (which crosses the placenta more readily).

Severe, acute attacks of migraine should be treated aggressively. We start IV fluids (D5 in one-half normal saline) for hydration and then use prochlorperazine 10 mg IV to control both nausea and head pain. IV opioids or IV corticosteroids can be used to supplement this treatment. This is an extremely effective way of handling status migrainosus during pregnancy.

Preventive Treatment

Increased frequency and severity of migraine associated with nausea and vomiting may justify the use of preventive medication. Consider preventive treatment when patients experience at least three or four prolonged, severe attacks a month that are particularly incapacitating or unresponsive to symptomatic therapy and may result in dehydration and fetal distress. β-Adrenergic blockers such as propranolol have been used, although adverse events, including intrauterine growth retardation, have been reported. If the migraine is so severe that drug treatment is essential, the patient should be told of the risks posed by all the drugs that are used. If the patient has a coexistent illness that requires treatment, pick one drug that will treat both disorders. For example, propranolol can be used to treat hypertension and migraine, and fluoxetine can be used to treat comorbid depression (Tables 7.13 and 7.14).

ERRATA

An error has been noticed in Table 7.13. The corrected table is shown below.

TABLE 7.13 Preventive Treatment—Antidepressants and Antiepileptic Drugs

	Fetal Risk	
	FDA	**TERIS**
Tricyclics		
Amitriptyline	C	Unl
Doxepin	C	U
Imipramine	C	Unl
Nortriptyline	C	U
Protriptyline	C	U
SSRI/SNRI		
Citalopram	C	U
Duloxitine	C	U
Fluoxetine	C	Unl
Paroxetine	C	Unl
Sertraline	B	Unl
Venlafaxine	C	U
AEDs		
Gabapentin	C	U
Topiramate	C	U
Valproic acid	D	Mod

TABLE 7.13 Preventive Treatment—Antidepressants and Antiepileptic Drugs

	Fetal Risk	
	FDA	TERIS
Tricyclics	C	Unl
Amitriptyline	C	U
Doxepin	C	Unl
Imipramine	C	U
Nortriptyline	C	U
Protriptyline		
Citalopram	C	U
Duloxitine	C	U
Fluoxetine	C	Unl
Paroxetine	C	Unl
Sertraline	B	Unl
Venlafaxine	C	U
Gabapentin	C	U
Topiramate	C	U
Valproic acid	C	Mod

TABLE 7.14 Preventive Treatment: β-Blockers and Calcium Channel Blockers

	Fetal Risk	
	FDA	TERIS
β-Blockers		
Atenolol	D	U
Metoprolol	C[a]	U
Nadolol	C[a]	U
Propranolol	C[a]	U
Timolol	C[a]	U
Calcium channel blockers		
Verapamil	C	U

[a] Second or third trimester.

Nonpharmacologic Therapy

Nonpharmacologic therapy is especially important in headache management during pregnancy. Behavior modification (e.g., avoiding migraine triggers) can be highly effective, especially when combined with other therapies.

Regular habits, such as regular sleep, exercise, meals, work habits, and time for relaxation, can reduce headache frequency. Patients should avoid sleeping-in, over-exercising, skipping meals, excess stress, becoming overtired, and over-using stimulants such as caffeine. They should be warned about the dangers of overusing acute treatments. This can result in increased headache frequency and may pose an additional risk to the fetus.

The most commonly used nonpharmacologic techniques are biofeedback, acupuncture, and physical therapy.

Drug Exposure

If a woman inadvertently takes a drug while she is pregnant or becomes pregnant while taking a drug, determine if the drug is a known teratogen (although for many drugs this is not possible) (Table 7.15).

TABLE 7.15 Drug Exposure

- Determine exposure(s) dose, timing, and duration
- Ascertain patient's past and present health
  - Presence of mental retardation or chromosomal abnormalities in family
- If drug is known teratogen or risk unknown
  - Confirm gestational age by ultrasound
- Exposure during embryogenesis
  - High resolution ultrasound can determine whether damage has occurred
  - If normal, then fetal structure normal (within 90% sensitivity)
- Have obstetrician discuss results of studies with mother and significant other
- Formal prenatal counseling may be helpful

REFERENCES

American College of Obstetrics and Gynecology Committee on Practice Bulletins-Gynecology. ACOG practice bulletin no. 73: use of hormonal contraception in women with coexisting medical conditions. *Obstet Gynecol.* 2006;107:1453–1472.

Silberstein SD. Headaches, pregnancy and lactation. In: Yankowitz J, Niebyl JR, eds. *Drug Therapy in Pregnancy*. 3rd ed. Philadelphia, PA: Lippincott Williams and Wilkins;2001:231–246.

Silberstein SD. Menstrual migraine. In: Silberstein SD, ed. *Sex Hormones and Headache*. Philadelphia, PA: Current Medicine Group;2007:67–88.

Silberstein SD. Migraine associated with hormonal contraceptive use. In: Silberstein SD, ed. *Sex Hormones and Headache*. Philadelphia, PA: Current Medicine Group;2007:89–108.

Silberstein SD, Elkind AH, Schreiber C, Keywood C. Randomized trial of fro-vatriptan for the intermittent prevention of menstrual migraine. *Neurology.* 2004;63:261–269.

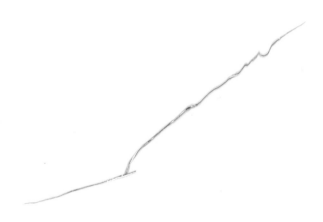

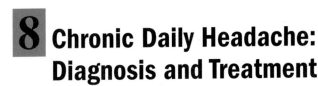 Chronic Daily Headache: Diagnosis and Treatment

INTRODUCTION

Chronic daily headache (CDH) refers to headache disorders in which attacks are experienced 15 or more days a month. Population-based studies suggest that 4% to 5% of the general population have primary CDH. In population samples, but not in the clinic, chronic tension-type headache (CTTH) is the leading cause of primary CDH (Table 8.1).

When the headache duration is less than 4 hours, the differential diagnosis includes cluster headache, paroxysmal hemicrania, idiopathic stabbing

TABLE 8.1 Primary CDH Sufferers Subdivided into Two Groups

- Paroxysmal headache
  - Duration <4 hours or multiple discrete episodes
- CDH
  - Daily or near-daily headache lasting ≥4 hours

Abbreviation: CDH, chronic daily headache.

TABLE 8.2 Primary and Secondary CDH

Primary CDH
- Headache duration ≥4 hours
  - Chronic migraine
  - Chronic tension-type headache
  - New daily persistent headache
  - Hemicrania continua

Secondary CDH
- Medication overuse headache
- Posttraumatic headache
- Cervical spine disorders
- Headache associated with vascular disorders (arteriovenous malformation, arteritis [including giant cell arteritis], dissection, and subdural hematoma)
- Headache associated with nonvascular intracranial disorders (intracranial hypertension, infection [Epstein-Barr virus, HIV], neoplasm)
- Other (temporomandibular joint disorder, sinus infection)

Abbreviations: CDH, chronic daily headache.

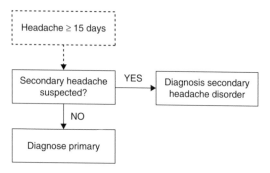

FIGURE 8.1 Clinical approach to CDH.

headache, hypnic headache, and short-lasting unilateral neuralgiform headache with conjunctival injection and tearing (SUNCT). When the headache duration is more than 4 hours, the major primary disorders to consider are chronic migraine (CM), hemicrania continua (HC), CTTH, and new daily persistent headache (NDPH) (Table 8.2 and Figure 8.1).

The new ICHD-II classification includes CM, which is similar, but not identical, to transformed migraine (TM). Silberstein and Lipton's criteria for TM provided three alternative diagnostic links to migraine (Table 8.3).

Migraine often transforms into CDH as a result of medication overuse, but transformation can occur without overuse. About 80% of CDH patients seen in subspecialty clinics overuse acute medication. The ICHD-II criteria for CM require that migraine or headache that responds to a triptan or ergot occurs at least 8 days a month and that headache is present at least 15 days a month (Table 8.4).

When medication overuse is present (and the headache worsens with overuse), medication overuse headache (MOH) is the diagnosis. MOH was previously called rebound headache, drug-induced headache, and medication-misuse headache. Medication overuse can make headaches refractory to preventive

TABLE 8.3 Silberstein-Lipton Criteria for Transformed Migraine

A. Daily or almost-daily (>15 days/month) head pain for >1 month
B. Average headache duration of >4 hours/day (if untreated)
C. At least one of the following:
  1. History of episodic migraine
  2. History of increasing headache frequency over at least 3 months
  3. Headache at some time meets International Headache Society criteria for migraine other than duration
D. Does not meet criteria for new daily persistent headache (4.7) or hemicrania continua (4.8)
E. Not attributable to another disorder

TABLE 8.4 ICHD-II Revised Criteria for Chronic Migraine

1. Headache (tension-type and/or migraine) on 15 or more days per month for at least 3 months
2. Five prior attacks of migraine without aura
3. On > 8 days per month for > 3 months headache
   Has fulfilled criteria for pain and associated symptoms of migraine without aura
   Treated and relieved by triptan(s) or ergots
4. No medication overuse and not attributed to another causative disorder

TABLE 8.5 ICHD-II Criteria for Headache Attributed to Medication Overuse

A. Headache present on >15 days/month
B. Regular overuse for > 3 months of one or more acute/symptomatic treatment drugs as defined under subforms of 8.2
   1. Ergotamine, triptans, opioids, or combination analgesic medications on ≥10 days/month on a regular basis for >3 months
   2. Simple analgesics or any combination of ergotamine, triptans, analgesics opioids on ≥ 15 days/month on a regular basis for > 3 months without overuse of any single class alone
C. Headache has developed or markedly worsened during medication overuse

medication. Although stopping the acute medication may result in withdrawal symptoms and a period of increased headache, subsequent headache improvement usually, but not always, occurs (Table 8.5).

Medication overuse is usually motivated by a patient's desire to treat his or her headaches. However, some patients with headache overuse combination analgesics containing butalbital to treat a mood disturbance.

DIFFERENTIATING CHRONIC MIGRAINE FROM OTHER CHRONIC DAILY HEADACHES

Chronic Tension-type Headache

CTTH requires head pain for 15 days a month for 3 months; many patients have daily headache. CTTH may develop in patients with a history of episodic tension-type headache. In this condition, headaches are often diffuse or bilateral and frequently involve the posterior aspect of the head and neck. In contrast to patients with CM, patients with CTTH do not have prior or coexistent episodic migraine, and most features of migraine are absent (Tables 8.6 and 8.7).

New Daily Persistent Headache

NDPH is characterized by the relatively abrupt onset of an unremitting primary CDH. NDPH is unique; the daily headache develops abruptly, over fewer

TABLE 8.6 CTTH Versus TM/CM

CTTH
■ Low-grade daily or almost-daily chronic headache *without* migrainous features
TM/CM
■ Daily or almost-daily headache *with* superimposed migrainous features
■ CM now accepted by It's IHS

Abbreviations: CM, chronic migraine; CTTH, chronic tension-type headache; IHS, International Headache Society; TM, transformed migraine.

TABLE 8.7 ICHD-II Criteria for Chronic Tension-type Headache

A. At least 10 episodes fulfilling criteria B-E. Number of days with such headache ≥15 days per month for at least 3 months period (=180 days per year).
B. Headache lasts hours or may be continuous
C. At least two of the following pain characteristics:
    1. Pressing or tightening quality
    2. Mild or moderate severity (may inhibit, but does not prohibit activities)
    3. Bilateral location
    4. No aggravation by walking stairs or similar routine physical activity
D. Both of the following:
    1. No more than one of the following: Photophobia, phonophobia, or mild nausea
    2. No moderate or severe nausea, and no vomiting
E. Not attributed to another disorder including medication overuse headache

than 3 days, and the patient typically has no prior headache history. It can continue for years without any sign of alleviation despite aggressive treatment. Patients with NDPH are generally younger than those with TM. The ICHD-II criteria limit NDPH to acute onset CTTH. We disagree and only agree with A, B, and E (Table 8.8).

NDPH can be extremely disabling. Many consider primary NDPH to be the most treatment-refractory of all headache disorders. NDPH patients often overuse medications, but, unlike patients with MOH, stopping the overuse does not relieve their pain. In contrast, the self-limited form of NDPH has a good prognosis, because patients appear to improve without any intervention.

NDPH, by definition, is not a secondary headache disorder, but patients often describe a flu-like illness or stressful life event as a trigger. Systemic infections, including Epstein-Barr virus, *Salmonella*, adenovirus, and herpes zoster, have been found in patients with NDPH. Since the publication of the ICHD-II criteria, several case series have described the clinical characteristics

TABLE 8.8 ICHD-II Criteria for New Daily Persistent Headache

A. Headache for >3 months fulfilling criteria B-D
B. Headache is daily and unremitting from onset or <3 days from onset
C. At least two of the following pain characteristics:
    1. Bilateral location
    2. Pressing/tightening (nonpulsating) quality
    3. Mild or moderate intensity
    4. Not aggravated by routine physical activity such as walking or climbing stairs
D. Both of the following
    1. No more than one of photophobia, phonophobia, or mild nausea
    2. Neither moderate/severe nausea nor vomiting
E. Not attributed to another disorder

of NDPH. The following statements are true of patients with NDPH:

■ Women are more commonly affected than men
■ Adolescents may be more commonly affected than adults
■ Many patients experience typical migraine symptoms
■ Comorbid disorders, such as depression, anxiety, fibromyalgia, and irritable bowel syndrome, have a prevalence similar to migraine
■ A family history of NDPH is rare, but migraine is common
■ Preventive medications used in other headache disorders may be helpful
■ Exclude secondary headache disorders with neuroimaging, lumbar puncture, and blood studies—especially in older patients

Hemicrania Continua

HC is an indomethacin-responsive headache disorder that is characterized by a continuous, moderately severe, unilateral headache that varies in intensity, waxing, and waning without disappearing completely. Exacerbations of pain are often associated with autonomic disturbances, such as ptosis, miosis, tearing, and sweating. Clinically, HC may alternate sides, although this is rare and is in contradiction to the ICHD-II criteria. In addition, some patients fulfill every criterion except indomethacin responsiveness, and how to classify such patients remains debatable (Table 8.9).

HC is more common than is currently believed and may present with relatively rapid onset. Associated symptoms can be divided into three main categories. These include autonomic symptoms, "jabs and jolts," and migrainous features (nausea, photophobia, phonophobia, or aura). Autonomic symptoms include conjunctival injection, tearing, rhinorrhea, nasal stuffiness, eyelid edema, a sense of aural fullness, and forehead sweating. Many patients note discomfort or a foreign body sensation in the eye. When present, photophobia

TABLE 8.9 ICHD-II Diagnostic Criteria for Hemicrania Continua

A. Headache for >3 months fulfilling criteria B-D
B. All of the following characteristics:
   1. Unilateral pain without side-shift
   2. Daily and continuous without pain-free periods
   3. Moderate intensity but with exacerbation of severe pain
C. At least one of the autonomic features occurs during exacerbation and ipsilateral to the side of pain.
   1. Conjunctival lacrimation and/or lacrimation
   2. Nasal congestion and/or rhinorrhea
   3. Ptosis and/or miosis
D. Complete response to therapeutic doses of indomethacin
E. Not attributed to another disorder

in HC is usually unilateral, unlike in most migraineurs. Autonomic symptoms are usually less prominent than in those with trigeminal autonomic cephalgias (TACs), and a few patients deny autonomic symptoms. Some patients experience an episodic form of HC with distinct headache phases followed by pain-free periods, and patients may change forms over time. Indomethacin is the mainstay of treatment, although there are case reports of patients responding to agents such as gabapentin, verapamil, topiramate, melatonin, occipital nerve blocks, and neurostimulator devices in patients with contraindications to, severe side effects from, or lack of improvement with indomethacin.

Patients with suspected HC should undergo investigation to rule out secondary causes and receive a course of indomethacin to make the diagnosis. Although recent case series suggest that HC may not be rare, unilateral side-locked migraine is common and many patients with a phenotype of HC do not respond to adequate doses of indomethacin. Some patients are able to reduce their indomethacin dose after successful treatment, but most will need to stay on the drug.

Secondary causes of HC are not rare and include the following:

■ Head trauma or postcraniotomy
■ Internal carotid artery aneurysm or dissection (Figure 8.2)
■ Vascular malformations (Figure 8.3)
■ Sphenoidal or pituitary tumor
■ Lung carcinoma
■ Postpartum

RISK FACTORS FOR CHRONIC DAILY HEADACHE

Significant risk factors for CDH include analgesic overuse, a history of migraine, and depression. At follow-up, patients with persistent primary CDH had a significantly higher frequency of analgesic overuse and major depression (Table 8.10).

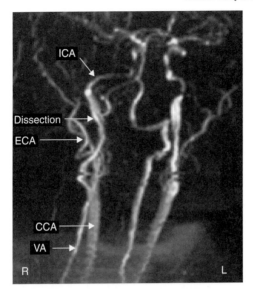

FIGURE 8.2 Right internal carotid dissection producing secondary HC.
Source: From Ashkenazi et al., *Headache,* 2007.

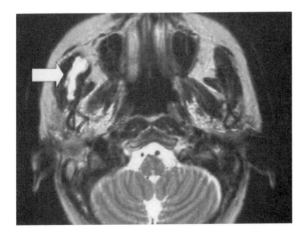

FIGURE 8.3 Venous malformation in the right masseter muscle producing secondary HC.
Source: From D'Alessio et al., *Cephalalgia,* 2004.

TABLE 8.10 Risk Factors for CDH

1. High headache frequency	7. Acute medication overuse
2. Female gender	8. Depression
3. Obesity (BMI > 30)	9. Head trauma
4. Snoring	10. History of migraine
5. Stressful life events	11. Less than a high school education
6. High caffeine consumption	

Abbreviation: BMI, body mass index; CDH, chronic daily headache.

CDH is more common in women, those previously married, those with obesity, and those with less education. Obesity, high baseline headache frequency, high caffeine consumption, snoring, and stressful life events were significantly associated with new-onset CDH.

TREATMENT

Patients should be started on preventive medication (to decrease reliance on acute medication) with the explicit understanding that the drugs may not become fully effective until medication overuse has been eliminated. Outpatient treatment in an ambulatory infusion unit and home treatment options are available. If outpatient treatment proves difficult or is dangerous, hospitalization may be required.

Patients can have severe exacerbations of their migraine during detoxification. Patients often need additional treatment (*headache terminators*) to break the cycle of CDH and/or help with the exacerbation that occurs when overused medications are discontinued. Withdrawal symptoms include severely exacerbated headaches accompanied by nausea, vomiting, agitation, restlessness, sleep disorder, and (rarely) seizures. Barbiturates, opioids, and benzodiazepines, unless replaced with long-acting derivatives, must be tapered to avoid an uncomfortable or serious withdrawal syndrome (Table 8.11).

TABLE 8.11 How to Manage Difficult-to-Treat CDH Patients

1. Exclude secondary headache
2. Diagnose CDH subtype: TM/CM, HC, CTTH, or NDPH
3. Identify coexistent conditions, especially MOH
4. Start preventive medication (may not work until overuse eliminated)
5. Limit acute medications
6. Some patients need their headache cycles terminated

Abbreviations: CDH, chronic daily headache; CM, chronic migraine; CTTH, chronic tension-type headache; HC, hemicrania continua; MOH, medication overuse headache; NDPH, new daily persistent headache; TM, transformed migraine.

Acute Pharmacotherapy

The choice of acute medication depends on the diagnosis. CM patients, who by definition are not overusing acute medication, can treat acute migrainous headache exacerbations with antimigraine drugs. These must be strictly limited to prevent MOH, which will complicate treatment and require detoxification (Chapter 9). CTTH and NDPH can be treated with nonspecific headache medications, and HC can be treated with supplemental doses of indomethacin.

Preventive Pharmacotherapy

The most widely used preventive drugs are tricyclic antidepressants, such as nortriptyline and amitriptyline, which are effective in many but not all studies. Fluoxetine and divalproex sodium may be effective, and β-blockers are also used. Gabapentin is mildly effective. Based on two randomized, placebo-controlled,

TABLE 8.12 Preventive Medications for Patients with Very Frequent or Daily Headaches

Drug	Clinical Efficacy	Adverse Events	Clinical Evidence*
Antidepressants			
Amitriptyline	+++	++	+++
Doxepin	+++	++	++
Fluoxetine	++	+	+++
Anticonvulsants			
Divalproex	+++	++	++
Gabapentin	++	++	+++
Topiramate	++++	++	+++
β-Blockers			
Propranolol, nadolol, etc.	++	+	+
Calcium channel blockers			
Verapamil	++	+	+
Neurotoxins			
Onabotulinum toxin A	++++	+	+++

*Ratings of +++ for clinical evidence indicate at least one double-blind, placebo-controlled study. A rating of ++ indicates open well-designed studies and + indicates ratings based on clinical experience. A rating of ++++ requires at least two double-blind, placebo-controlled trials.
For doses, see Chapter 9.

double-blind, parallel-group, multicenter studies, topiramate (100 mg/day) is effective in CM even in the presence of medication overuse.

Although monotherapy is preferred, it is sometimes necessary to combine preventive medications. Antidepressants are often used with β-blockers or calcium channel blockers, and divalproex sodium may be used in combination with any of these medications (Table 8.12).

Neurotoxins
New placebo-controlled trials have shown that injection with onabotulinum toxin A is effective in CM even in the presence of medication overuse. Based on data from phase 3 double-blind, placebo-controlled trials, patients receiving onabotulinum toxin A, 155 to 195 units given at 31 to 39 sites, had significantly fewer migraine and headache days and reduced acute medication use. Common injection sites include procerus, corrugators, frontalis, temporalis, occipitalis, splenius capitus, cervical paraspinals, sternocleidomastoid, and trapezius muscles (Figure 8.4).

REFERENCES

Goadsby PJ, Lipton RB. A review of paroxysmal hemicranias, SUNCT syndrome and other short-lasting headaches with autonomic features, including new cases. *Brain*. 1997;120:193–209.

Headache Classification Committee. The International Classification of Headache Disorders: 2nd ed. *Cephalalgia*. 2004;24:1–160.

Scher AI, Stewart WF, Ricci JA, Lipton RB. Factors associated with the onset and remission of chronic daily headache in a population-based study. *Pain*. 2003;106:89.

Silberstein SD, Lipton RB, Saper JR. Chronic daily headache including transformed migraine, chronic tension-type headache, and medication overuse headache. In: Silberstein SD, Lipton RB, Dodick DW, eds. *Wolff's Headache and Other Head Pain*. 8th ed. New York, NY: Oxford University Press;2007:315–378.

Zwart JA, Dyb G, Hagen K, Svebak S, Holmen J. Analgesic use: a predictor of chronic pain and medication overuse headache: the Head-HUNT Study. *Neurology*. 2003;61:160–164.

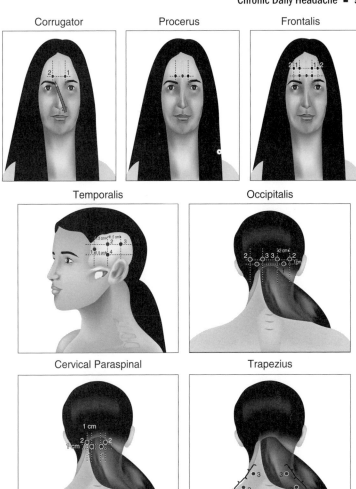

FIGURE 8.4 Selected onabotulinum toxin A injection sites.

Medication Overuse: Diagnosis and Treatment

INTRODUCTION

Medication overuse can cause or complicate chronic daily headache (CDH). When overuse is the cause of CDH, it is termed medication overuse headache (MOH).

Other names for this disorder include rebound headache and drug-induced headache. Over time (defined in treatment days per month, with a variable threshold depending on the substance overused), frequent acute headache medication use tends to perpetuate or aggravate an existing headache disorder in a susceptible individual, and often renders preventive medication ineffective. MOH is quite common, and in specialty clinics patients may account for the vast majority of the treatment population (Tables 9.1 and 9.2).

TABLE 9.1 Medication Overuse Headache (Composite ICHD-II Criteria)

A. Headache present on ≥15 days/month
B. Regular overuse for >3 months of ≥1 acute/symptomatic treatment drugs[a]
   1. Ergotamine, triptans, opioids, or combination analgesic medications on ≥10 days/month on a regular basis for >3 months
   2. Simple analgesics on ≥15 days/month on a regular basis for > 3 months
   3. Intake of any combination of acute medications on ≥15 days/month for >3 months without overuse of any single class alone
C. Headache has developed or markedly worsened during medication overuse

[a] Substances used for other pain conditions, or for recreational purposes, affect MOH and "count toward" treatment days.

TABLE 9.2 MOH Prevalence

- In European headache centers
  - 5% to 10% of patients
- In Italian headache centers
  - 4.3% of 3000 consecutive patients
- In specialty headache clinics
  - 50% to 80% of CDH patients
- In US population
  - 28% of CM patients
- CDH seven times more likely to develop with MOH than without

Abbreviations: CDH, chronic daily headache; CM, chronic migraine; MOH, medication overuse headache.

MOH should be distinguished from addiction, wherein patients experience cravings for and subsequently abuse substances with acute psychoactive properties for personal gratification despite repeated negative consequences of these actions. In contrast, MOH is a pseudoaddiction: patients are driven by a need for pain relief, but still use substances repeatedly, despite negative consequences. However, true addiction may coincide with MOH, especially when the overused medication contains an opioid or butalbital, thus making management even more complicated (Table 9.3).

As with all headache disorders, a systematic approach to diagnosis and treatment yields the best chances for success.

TABLE 9.3 MOH—Drugs Implicated

High probability	Possibly
Opioids	Aspirin
Ergotamine	Acetaminophen
Butalbital	NSAIDs
Caffeine	Unlikely
Triptans	Neuroleptics
	DHE

Abbreviations: DHE, dihydroergotamine; MOH, medication overuse headache; NSAIDs, nonsteroidal anti-inflammatory drugs.

ASSESSMENT

All patients with CDH must be assessed for MOH. Most patients and many physicians are unaware of the concept, and in fact, some patients have developed MOH after getting bad advice from their physicians. Only a few patients will recognize the problem on their own and initiate the discussion with their doctor.

Questions to Ask

1. How many days each month do you have any kind of headache?
2. How many days each month do you take something, *anything*, to relieve your headaches? (Don't forget about over-the-counter or "alternative" treatments)
3. What do you take, how much, and under what circumstances (e.g., mild/moderate/severe, at work vs. at home, "when you just can't take it anymore," etc.)?
4. Do you find yourself taking pain medication to prevent a headache before it has even really started, or because you fear developing a headache? How often?
5. Do you find yourself taking medication compulsively, even when it isn't really effective?

6. Do you take any other pain medications for any other conditions? What? How often?
7. How much caffeine do you take in on an average day?
8. Do you ever use any substances for recreational purposes? How often?
9. Do you have an "addictive personality," or have you ever had problems refraining from habitual nonproductive behavior like smoking, drug/alcohol misuse, gambling, excessive sexual behavior, excessive spending, and the like?

Calendars

Some patients will not be able to tell you how often their headaches occur or about all their behaviors. This is why calendars are essential to document headache (and other pain) patterns and substance use. Giving a patient a pre-printed calendar with fields for headache intensity/duration, treatment taken, and response to treatment greatly improves adherence.

ACUTE PHASE TREATMENT

It is essential not only to recognize MOH but also to diagnose the underlying primary headache problem, as this affects treatment decisions (e.g., the patient may have as-yet undiagnosed hemicrania continua). Comorbid/coexistent conditions must be ascertained. Ask what preventive agents the patient has tried. Although the trial may have failed, it may be worth repeating (unless there was a safety or tolerability issue) as MOH may render preventive medications ineffective. Some patients with MOH improve simply by removing the offending medication(s); some will not, and most, in their pre-MOH state, would have been considered appropriate for and in need of preventive treatment. Since preventive medication takes weeks if not months to work, it should be initiated sooner rather than later (Table 9.4).

TABLE 9.4 MOH Treatment—Initial Approach

■ Diagnose the primary underlying CDH subtype: transformed/chronic migraine, hemicrania continua, chronic tension-type headache, new daily persistent headache
■ Identify comorbid/coexistent conditions
■ Start tailored preventive treatment (may not work until overuse eliminated)
■ Initiate detoxification (triptans, ergotamine, and simple analgesics easier than opioids, barbiturates, or combination drugs)
■ Attempt to terminate the headache cycle

Abbreviations: CDH, chronic daily headache; MOH, medication overuse headache.

The overused agent(s) can be removed in a number of ways. A conservative, simple approach is to give the patient a schedule to taper his or her pain medications with a "quit date," but this can take quite some time, and the quit date may be postponed again and again as the patient fails to abstain from treatment because of a need to function and be free from severe pain. Neuroleptics or corticosteroids can be useful short-term adjuncts in managing increased pain levels and keeping the patient away from the old medications.

Substitution is another approach. For example, if an opioid is overused, give the patient a long-acting one, such as methadone (which can be of additional benefit because of its NMDA-receptor effects), with instructions to taper over time. Use an opioid dose conversion calculator (many are available free online), and compute a 50% dose reduction for cross-tolerance. This ensures that the patient is not overdosed on the new opioid and also reduces the ground that must be covered on the road to abstinence. Some patients have difficulty managing opioid withdrawal symptoms, which may be unpredictable in their timing. Some find it easier with concomitant treatment with clonidine (0.1–0.3 mg once or twice daily, or a weekly patch, blood pressure permitting) and/ or benzodiazepines (either standing low-dose clonazepam or prn lorazepam; benzodiazepines should be tapered as well to avoid a potentially harmful withdrawal syndrome). Other substitutions include dihydroergotamine (DHE) for triptans (patients must be trusted not to take triptans while using DHE), and phenobarbital for butalbital-containing medications. An approximate conversion is 30 mg phenobarbital per 100 mg of butalbital (most butalbital-containing medicines have 50 mg butalbital per tablet). Plan to taper butalbital over several days to a few weeks, depending on the total amount given (Table 9.5).

TABLE 9.5 Outpatient Detoxification Strategies

- Give patient a schedule with daily intake limits to taper off overused medication
- Substitute a similar medication and taper it
  - DHE instead of triptan
  - Methadone instead of other opioids (use a conversion calculator and compute at least 50% dose reduction for cross-tolerance)
  - Phenobarbital instead of butalbital-containing combination analgesic (approximate conversion of 30 mg phenobarbital per 100 mg butalbital)
- While tapering, provide a compatible adjunctive treatment, such as a neuroleptic or corticosteroid
- Ensure that counseling for addiction/pseudoaddiction, compulsive drug-taking, anxiety, and so on occurs regularly throughout detoxification process

Abbreviation: DHE, dihydroergotamine.

A "bridge" approach is another method that may be tried. This may work better in the absence of opioid or butalbital overuse, because no dangerous or uncomfortable withdrawal syndrome occurs with abrupt discontinuation of other agents. In this approach, patients are strictly forbidden from using their preferred medication and instead are given a combination of new drugs to use over several days. This usually involves anti-inflammatory medication (steroidal or nonsteroidal), neuroleptic medication (for nausea as well as headache), and DHE (intranasal or intramuscular). The concept is that the patient will "blast" the headache and "break" it with these new medications, and thereafter use them appropriately, with limits, to manage headaches more effectively (Table 9.6).

TABLE 9.6 Some Bridge Examples

1. Day 1+2: prednisone 60 mg in the morning, prochlorperazine 10 mg (and Migranal four sprays tid prn)
   Day 3+4: prednisone 40 mg, prochlorperazine 10 mg bid/tid (and Migranal four sprays bid prn)
   Day 5+6: prednisone 20 mg, prochlorperazine 10 mg once/tid (and Migranal four sprays once prn)
   Day 7+8: prochlorperazine up to tid prn
2. For 4 days: naproxen sodium 550 mg plus metoclopramide 10 mg tid (and DHE 1 mg IM bid prn)
3. Dexamethasone qam tapering from 20 mg to zero over 5 days with olanzapine 10 to 20 mg qhs and tapering to zero over 7 days

Abbreviation: DHE, dihydroergotamine.

Finally, a biobehavioral treatment plan must be initiated. Educate the patient about nonpharmacologic treatment approaches. These could be as simple as distraction, rest, ice, heat, or massage. More sophisticated means of managing headaches without medication include meditation, deep breathing exercises, guided imagery exercises, and biofeedback. These require training and practice to become effective. Many patients harbor a great deal of anxiety. They may fear that their next attack will be particularly disabling or interfere with an important planned event. Some patients catastrophize so much that they may actually cause themselves to develop a headache. Some patients have frank issues of addiction or drug abuse. For these reasons, psychological referral, preferably to a practitioner with particular expertise in addiction or pain, is often warranted. The behavioral approach may also entail regimentation of the patient's day-to-day life. Mandating regular sleep schedules, frequent small healthful meals, and an aerobic conditioning program are just a few simple but important means of helping to restore health and functioning.

If the aforementioned measures fail, if it is considered unsafe or likely futile to treat on an outpatient basis, or if faster results are needed or desired, this process should be carried out in the inpatient setting. There are several advantages to this approach. Detoxification can be achieved more rapidly and safely. Intravenous fluids, in the initial phase, speed washout of undesirable drugs and substances. In a monitored setting, withdrawal syndromes were managed more efficiently due to more regular, personalized contact with the clinical team. Symptomatic medication, rather than supplemental doses of the medication being eliminated, can be used aggressively to quicken the process, and moreover, the use of high-potency parenteral medication for headache and associated symptoms aids in keeping the patient more comfortable during what is often a very difficult transition. Hospitalization for detoxification is not only safer and faster but also carries a higher likelihood for success in such a controlled setting (Table 9.7).

TABLE 9.7 Inpatient Detoxification Strategies

- When outpatient detoxification fails or is not safe
- Generally allows for faster, safer detoxification
    - Intravenous fluids to speed washout
    - Rapid detoxification, efficient management of withdrawal
    - Concomitant high-potency parenteral headache medications
    - Controlled setting increases safety and chance of success

It is important to remember that not all patients will improve within the expected timeframe of several weeks to a few months of restricted abortive medication use. This does not mean that excessive use of pain medication was not a factor in the initiation or maintenance of CDH, and it does not mean that the patient should return to the habit of treating frequently with abortives in an effort to maintain control and preserve functioning. Rather, preventive treatment modalities must be pursued more aggressively, and after these strategies have been implemented, repeated attempts at terminating the pattern of continuous or recurrent headaches should be undertaken. Unfortunately, some patients are medically refractory and never seem to improve. Again, this is no reason to liberalize abortive use, but rather continue exploring new preventive strategies, and make ongoing efforts to reduce medication load in general (e.g., sleep aids, stimulants, multiple medications with overlapping purposes) as these medications could have unrecognized effects on headaches(Table 9.8).

TABLE 9.8 Recommended Limits for Specific Acute Medications to Prevent MOH

- Ergot, triptan, or simple combination analgesics
  - Limit to 8 days/month
- Butalbital-containing analgesics (e.g., Fioricet) and opioids
  - Limit to 5 days/month (men may be OK taking butalbital up to 8 days/month, and women may be OK taking opioids up to 8 days/month)
- Other analgesics
  - Limit to 12 days/month
- Total exposure
  - Limit to 12 days/month

Abbreviations: MOH, medication overuse headache.
These are less than the definition of MOH, a buffer is included.

LONG-TERM TREATMENT

Use headache calendars to monitor patient progress. Encourage patients to use and document nonmedication treatment (rest in a dark quiet room, ice/heat, massage, distraction, meditation, or other relaxation techniques) for every attack, because these measures can be effective on their own and can enhance acute medication effect. This also gives patients the opportunity to explore novel nonmedication therapies and practice their relaxation strategies.

In the long-term plan, reassess acute and preventive medications. Ensure that acute medications continue to be used appropriately, that they are effective, and that they are not associated with adverse events. For example, triptans or DHE are not appropriate for patients with increased risk for cardiovascular or cerebrovascular disease: these risks must be ascertained and reassessed over time. Frequent use of neuroleptic medication can lead to hyperlipidemia, glucose intolerance, weight gain, and tardive dyskinesia. Preventive medications also need to be monitored for safety and appropriateness. Sometimes preventive medication can be withdrawn slowly without CDH recurrence. Remember that CDH is a relapsing-remitting disorder, and preventive medication may need to be increased or new drugs introduced. Just because a patient begins to do poorly on a particular preventive medication regimen does not mean it should be scrapped entirely, but rather, fine-tuned. There are often mitigating circumstances associated with relapses (unidentified or undisclosed acute medication overuse, stress, medical illness, dietary indiscretion, nonadherence to lifestyle modification, etc.) which, when remedied, will result in return of control (Table 9.9).

TABLE 9.9 MOH Pearls

- Preventive treatment without withdrawal may be effective
- Full benefit of preventive drug takes 6 months
- Combination preventive treatment may be necessary
- CM and MOH are relapsing-remitting disorders
  - Long-term prevention is often necessary
  - Relapse does not always mean tachyphylaxis
- Set realistic expectations regarding outcomes
  - Mild daily headache with fewer exacerbations
  - Headache free
- Some patients are medically intractable and do not improve

Abbreviations: CM, chronic migraine; MOH, medication overuse headache.

REFERENCES

Andrasik F, Buse DC, Grazzi L. Behavioral medicine for migraine and medication overuse headache. *Curr Pain Headache Rep.* 2009;13(3):241–248.

Bigal ME, Lipton RB. Overuse of acute migraine medications and migraine chronification. *Curr Pain Headache Rep.* 2009;13(4):301–307.

Bigal ME, Serrano D, Buse D, Scher A, Stewart WF, Lipton RB. Acute migraine medications and evolution from episodic to chronic migraine: a longitudinal population-based study. *Headache.* 2008;48(8):1157–1168.

Rossi P, Jensen R, Nappi G, Allena M. A narrative review on the management of medication overuse headache: the steep road from experience to evidence. *J Headache Pain.* 2009;10(6):407–417.

Vargas BB, Dodick DW. The face of chronic migraine: epidemiology, demographics, and treatment strategies. *Neurol Clin.* 2009;27(2):467–479.

10 Comorbid Disorders Associated with Migraine and Chronic Daily Headache

Comorbidity was originally defined as the presence of any coexistent condition in a patient with an index disease. The currently accepted definition is an association between two disorders that is more than coincidental. Comorbidity may arise by coincidence or selection bias, or one condition may cause the other. Conditions may be related due to shared environmental or genetic risk factors, producing a brain state that gives rise to both conditions. Studies indicate that many disorders are comorbid with migraine (Table 10.1).

TABLE 10.1 Migraine Comorbidities

- Cardiovascular
  - Raynaud's phenomenon
  - Myocardial infarction
  - Ischemic stroke, subclinical stroke, white matter abnormalities
  - Patent foramen ovale (with aura)
  - Mitral valve prolapse
  - Atrial septal aneurysm
- Neurologic
  - Epilepsy
  - Restless legs syndrome
  - Vestibular disorders
  - Essential tremor?
- Psychiatric
  - Depression
  - Anxiety
  - Bipolar disorder
  - Panic disorder
  - Suicide risk
  - Phobia
- Others
  - Snoring/sleep apnea
  - Asthma/allergy
  - SLE
  - Non-headache pain
    - Fibromyalgia
    - Irritable bowel syndrome

Abbreviation: SLE, systemic lupus erythematosus.

PSYCHIATRIC COMORBIDITY

When Harold Wolff published the first edition of *Headache and Other Head Pain* in 1948, he (and others) believed that migraineurs were perfectionistic and obsessive, and this was the reason they suffered from migraine headaches. This original impression has not been borne out, and what has emerged is that

TABLE 10.2 Disorders Comorbid with Migraine

Diagnoses	Odds Ratio
Major depression	2.2–3.14
Bipolar spectrum	2.9
Any anxiety disorder	2.7
Panic disorder	3.0–5.09
Generalized anxiety disorder	5.3–5.5
Agoraphobia	2.4–2.5
Social phobia	1.45–3.4

Note: Comorbid association is generally higher with chronic than with episodic migraine.

migraine is comorbid with a number of Axis-I diagnoses. Table 10.2 shows migraineurs' population-based odds of having each of the comorbid psychiatric disorders, compared with nonmigraineurs.

The lifetime prevalence of these disorders is more in migraineurs than in nonmigraineurs, although the odds ratios (ORs) are less dramatic. This suggests that a migraineur with one of the aforementioned disorders has it more often or for longer than a nonmigraineur with psychiatric disease.

There is a stronger relationship between migraine with aura and the Axis-I diagnoses. The ratio is particularly large for bipolar and panic disorders, wherein migraineurs with aura have at least twice the risk as migraineurs without aura (Figure 10.1).

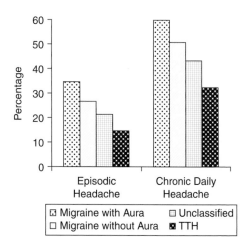

FIGURE 10.1 Depression risk of chronic versus episodic migraine patients.
Source: Frequent Headache Epidemiology Study.

Many patients have a distinctive time sequence: anxiety first, with an average age of onset of 12 years; migraine next, with onset at age 14; and depression last, with onset around 17 years of age. There is also a bidirectional influence between migraine and depression, and migraine and panic disorder. Individuals with migraine without depression are almost 5.8 times more likely to develop depression than those without migraine, and those with depression without migraine are 3.5 times more likely to develop migraine than those without depression. Panic disorder has a similar bidirectional relationship with migraine and is also a risk factor for increased migraine frequency.

Migraine with (but not without) aura is associated with a high risk of suicidal ideation and suicide attempts. Adolescents with chronic daily headache with aura have a high risk of suicide.

Migraineurs should be screened for psychiatric diseases. Migraine with aura and chronic daily headache appear to be independent risk factors for psychiatric disease, and aura is associated with suicide.

PAINFUL DISORDERS

Pain conditions often co-occur. These painful disorders include irritable bowel syndrome, headache, fibromyalgia, and other musculoskeletal pain. In clinic-based studies, migraine has been associated with fibromyalgia and irritable bowel syndrome. Cross-sectional associations show an association between migraine and chronic musculoskeletal pain (OR ≈ 1.8). The association is stronger for chronic daily headache of any headache type (women: OR = 5.3, men: OR = 3.6).

Migraine and Restless Legs Syndrome

The prevalence of restless legs syndrome (RLS) is higher in headache patients (especially migraineurs) than in nonheadache patients (17–22% vs 8–6%). Intractable migraine patients have a high RLS frequency (34%), and there is a familial concordance of migraine with aura and RLS. Persons with migraine and RLS may be at increased risk for neuroleptic-induced akathisia.

Migraine and Epilepsy

A number of factors suggest a link between migraine and epilepsy. Head trauma increases the risk of both disorders. Seizures can produce headache. Several epilepsy genes predispose to migraine. Familial hemiplegic migraine genes increase seizure risk. Migraine and epilepsy may be linked by brain hyperexcitability because of genetic or environmental risk factors. Migralepsy, in which an epileptic seizure arises in the course of a typical migraine aura, is rare but does occur.

Those with epilepsy are 2.4 times more likely to develop migraine than are their nonepileptic relatives. This relationship is independent of age of onset, classification or type of seizure (partial vs generalized), or etiology (idiopathic, head trauma, or other). The relatives of epilepsy patients are also 2.4 times more likely to develop migraine than the nonepileptic control group.

Migraine and Stroke

Both migraine and stroke may be associated with cerebral blood flow changes, focal neurologic deficits, and headache. Stroke may produce or trigger headaches, which may be ictal, preictal, or postictal. Prolonged migraine aura may produce stroke, which is true migrainous infarction.

Welch has divided migraine stroke into four categories:

1. Coexisting stroke and migraine
2. Stroke with clinical features of migraine
   - Symptomatic migraine
   - Migraine mimic
3. Migraine-induced stroke
   - Without risk factors
   - With risk factors
4. Uncertain

Two recent studies have confirmed the findings of case-control and cohort studies: migraine is associated with stroke in women of younger age, more so with aura, and the risks are increased exponentially with smoking and the use of oral contraceptives (Figure 10.2).

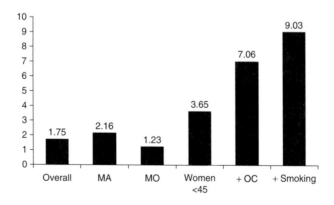

FIGURE 10.2 Risk of stroke in women with migraine. Odds ratio of having stroke. *Source*: Schurks *BMJ*, 2009.

TABLE 10.3 Risk of Transient Ischemic Attack and Stroke in Migraine

	Overall	Migraine with Aura	Migraine without Aura
Transient Ischemic Attack	OR =1.92[a] (1.50–2.47)	OR=3.36[a] (2.54–4.44)	OR = 1.21 (0.99–1.62)
Stroke	OR =1.54[a] (1.16–2.05)	OR=2.78[a] (2.02–3.84)	OR = 0.97 (0.69–1.36)

[a] Odds ratio with 95% confidence interval for transient ischemic attack and stroke compared to controls.

The American migraine prevalence and prevention study (AMPP) found that the risk that migraine confers for transient ischemic attack and stroke is limited to migraine with aura (Table 10.3).

Migraine and Coronary Artery Disease

In the AMPP study, migraineurs were 2.9 (with aura) and 1.9 (without aura) times the risk of developing myocardial infarction. Results were less robust in a large epidemiologic study of women, and significant only for migraine with aura.

CLINICAL IMPLICATIONS OF COMORBIDITY

The increased risk of having or developing a psychiatric illness implies that patients with migraine or chronic daily headache should be routinely surveyed for psychiatric disorders; in particular, these patients should be surveyed for suicide risk. Patients with major comorbid psychiatric disorders may require ongoing care with a mental health professional. We believe that some patients with severe anxiety or depression cannot be managed unless both headache and anxiety or depression are simultaneously addressed.

Patients with migraine and an excessive risk of cardiovascular disease should not be given ergotamines or triptans. There is little consensus about how many risk factors, at what age, constitute relative and absolute contraindications to triptan use, and when to stop prescribing triptans as a patient ages and accumulates cardiac risk factors while having demonstrable benefits in quality of life from triptan use. The frequent use of NSAIDs or Cox-2 inhibitors may increase the cardiovascular risk. If RLS is present, neuroleptics may be relatively contraindicated.

REFERENCES

Breslau N, Davis GC. Migraine, physical health and psychiatric disorders: a prospective epidemiologic study of young adults. *J Psychiatric Res.* 1993;27(2):211–221.

Breslau N, Schultz LR, Stewart WF, Lipton RB, Welch KM. Headache types and panic disorder: directionality and specificity. *Neurology.* 2001;56(3):350–354.

Kurth T, Gaziano JM, Cook NR, Logroscino G, Diener HC, Buring JE. Unreported financial disclosures in a study of migraine and cardiovascular disease. *JAMA.* 2006;296(6):653–654.

Schürks M, Rist PM, Bigal ME, Buring JE, Lipton RB, Kurth T. Migraine and cardiovascular disease: systematic review and metaanalysis. *BMJ.* 2009;339:3914.

Silberstein SD, Freitag FG, Bigal ME. Migraine diagnosis and comorbidity. In: Silberstein SD, Lipton RB, Dodick DW, eds. *Wolff's headache and Other Head Pain.* New York, NY: Oxford University press;2008:153–176.

11 Behavioral Treatment of Migraine and Chronic Daily Headache

INTRODUCTION

Some patients are able to manage their migraine with just lifestyle modification and behavioral approaches. Most patients, even if they need more than behavioral therapy alone, find that their acute and preventive medications become more effective when they use these techniques. They may not be appropriate for every patient; thus an individualized, tailored treatment plan is essential.

RELAXATION TRAINING

Patients with migraine often have some degree of anxiety. It may be a comorbid condition, or anxiety may revolve entirely around fears of the effect of migraine attacks. Stress can trigger migraine and generally adversely affects its management. Relaxation techniques are useful in reducing the effect of stress. Most of these techniques can be learned from a book (often accompanied by a tape, CD, or DVD), but one-on-one training by a licensed professional is preferable.

The simplest relaxation exercise is deep breathing. In a quiet atmosphere and relaxed position, the patient concentrates on breathing slowly and deeply, focusing on the movement of air and the abdominal muscles, and clearing the mind of all other thoughts. This should be done for several minutes, until full relaxation of body and mind is achieved.

Sequential muscle relaxation is often combined with deep breathing. Patients focus on individual muscles or small groups of them, and slowly, from head to toe, relax each one in sequence, taking several minutes to complete the exercise. Some patients find it helpful to then sequentially tighten the muscles, from toe to head, and even to do multiple cycles of relaxation and tightening.

Guided imagery is another technique that again can be utilized on its own or in conjunction with the aforementioned techniques. Until the patient is proficient doing this on his/her own, the practitioner, in person or via audio recording, guides the patient through imagined tranquil landscapes and sequences, such as a beach or rain forest. Again, the patient frees the mind of all intrusive thoughts and concentrates only on the relaxing beauty of the imagery. A dream-like state can be induced, and the patient can interact with the imagined environment to enhance the relaxation effect. The patient may imagine unrolling a blanket to place on the warm sand, gently massaging sunscreen over his/her body, then lying down to enjoy the soothing sunshine while simultaneously breathing deeply and practicing sequential muscle relaxation. These imagined sequences become quite vivid with practice, and eventually the patient can accomplish this without the aid of another person guiding the process.

Meditation

With meditation, the mind is more active, but the body remains relaxed. The patient enters a state of reflection, again in a quiet atmosphere free of interruptions. Some patients will use an anchoring code word, repeated over and over in the mind as a focus point, while simultaneously undergoing self-exploration. Others set aside time each morning to formulate the day's goals and how to achieve them, followed by an evening reflection on how well the goals were accomplished and how to obtain greater success in the future. Prayer can be incorporated into meditative exercises.

Hypnosis

Hypnosis is not commonly used but is very helpful to some patients. This is initiated with the aid of a professional, but some patients eventually learn self-hypnosis. There are similarities to guided imagery, but a specific objective of hypnosis is to uncover unconscious processes that underlie distress and dysfunction of the mind and body, and then restructure them to be productive toward self-improvement.

Cognitive-Behavioral Therapy

This is a fully conscious exploration of the interplay of thought and action directed by an experienced mental health professional. The focus is on identifying aberrant, counterproductive, or destructive thoughts and behaviors, remaining cognizant of them, and taking active measures to remedy them. A simple example may be the patient who is trying to quit smoking and does not recognize that some unfulfilled need in his or her personal life drives the desire to smoke. When the urge to smoke again is satisfied, guilt ensues, but the patient begins to rationalize that as long as a failure of will has occurred, there is no extra harm in continuing to smoke. Since what's done is done, he/she might as well enjoy smoking for the rest of the day and try quitting again the next day. Failures of this nature only set up future failures of the same sort, until this irrational cycle of thought and behavior is addressed.

Biofeedback

Ordinarily unconscious biological processes, such as regulation of heart rate, blood pressure, skin temperature, and muscle tone, can become modifiable with biofeedback training. The biological parameters are monitored and projected on a real-time display. The patient focuses on the display and attempts to modify the output. Achieving this skill requires dedication and practice, but once learned, it can be used effectively to manage stress, and some patients find that practicing this exercise can even abort a headache. Biofeedback is perhaps the best studied and most proven behavioral treatment modality in the management of headache.

Diet

Many "migraine diets" are touted, but there is scant hard, scientific evidence to support them. In general, we recommend a healthful, balanced diet. Low caffeine consumption and avoidance of excess alcohol, nitrates, and monosodium glutamate are good recommendations for most migraineurs. Probably of greater importance is adherence to a diet conducive to achieving and maintaining a normal body mass index, as we have learned that being either underweight or obese imparts risk for chronification of migraine.

Exercise

There is limited evidence that exercise benefits headache directly, but regular and varied physical activity helps the patient not only maintain weight control but also improve energy levels, promote better sleep, reduce stress, and alleviate body pains and muscle aches (e.g., fibromyalgia). Of course, there are barriers to initiating an exercise program, most notably the will to begin and continue, as well as the problem that exercise can sometimes trigger a migraine attack. Counsel patients to begin with something very simple and advance gradually as tolerated. Even if the initial step is only brisk walking for 10 minutes once or twice a week, it is a starting point. Patients need to set realistic goals and make exercise part of their daily or weekly routine, eventually working towards a goal of exercising for 20 to 30 minutes three times a week, and later advancing to a loftier goal of 60 minutes or more 5 to 7 days a week. A variety of exercises, such as aerobic conditioning, strength training, and stretching, is essential to a well-rounded program. Yoga is excellent, because it incorporates stretching, strength training, and relaxation techniques. For patients hampered by headaches triggered by cardiovascular workouts, suggest pretreatment with a nonsteroidal anti-inflammatory drug (NSAID) or even a triptan as appropriate.

Sleep

There is tremendous interplay between sleep and migraine. Sleep alone can relieve a migraine, but migraines can interfere with sleep. Many migraine patients complain of insomnia at night and sleepiness during the day. Disruption of sleep often triggers headache. Therefore, maintenance of regular sleep/wake schedules and good sleep-related behavior (i.e., sleep hygiene) is essential. Before using night-time sleep aids and daytime stimulants, educate patients about good sleep hygiene practices. Remind them that regular exercise, a relaxation program, and a healthful diet all promote better sleep (Table 11.1).

TABLE 11.1 Recommendations for Good Sleep Hygiene Practices

1. Get up in the morning and go to bed at night at the same time every day, even if you are very tired in the morning or not very sleepy at night
2. Do not nap during the day, no matter how tired you feel
3. Do not try to "catch up" on lost sleep during the weekend or off days by sleeping in
4. Avoid caffeine in the afternoon and evening
5. Avoid vigorous exercise later in the day
6. Avoid eating late in the evening
7. Do not drink alcohol excessively, or to help you sleep
8. Have a bedtime routine to help get your mind and body prepared for sleep
9. Your bed is only for sleeping (and sex, if you are sexually active). Do not engage in other leisure activities in bed, and if possible, not even in the bedroom itself. Sticking to this will condition your mind and body to associate sleep with your bed more strongly
10. Do not constantly watch the clock and worry about not falling asleep as time passes
11. If you don't fall asleep after 20 minutes, get up and do something nonstimulating for 10 to 15 minutes, then try again to fall asleep

Avoidance of Triggers

What are true migraine triggers? Many are perceived, but few are substantiated with scientific evidence. A recent prospective study utilizing sophisticated statistical analyses of detailed diary data identified factors, such as stress, lack of exercise, low atmospheric pressure, and sunshine more than 3 hours per day, that may increase the risk of migraine and serve as triggers. Tiredness and muscle tension also predict the occurrence of headache, although these may represent dopaminergic prodromal phenomena. Interestingly, this study showed reduced risk of headache with divorce, progesterone-only contraception, and beer consumption. No influence was seen from chocolate, cheese, nuts, red wine, cigarette smoke, other odors, hunger, or sleep disturbances—all commonly perceived headache triggers. It must, of course, be remembered that absence of evidence is not evidence of absence. Patients may have consciously avoided these potential precipitants, thus masking their contribution. Additionally, triggers can be highly individual-specific.

What about chocolate, the oft-maligned treat that is shunned by many a migraineur? It has been suggested that biogenic amines in chocolate may provoke headache, that the caffeine in chocolate may play a role, or that eating chocolate prior to a headache may merely be a hypothalamically driven migraine prodromal craving. A double-blind controlled study showed that chocolate is no more likely to trigger migraine than carob.

The multitude of potential migraine triggers, real and perceived, should be discussed in detail. Once a patient's true and false triggers are identified, he or she can avoid precipitants whenever possible and may regain pleasure from formerly avoided circumstances or substances.(Table 11.2)

TABLE 11.2   Cognitive and Behavioral Treatment Recommendations (AAN Practice Parameter)

- Relaxation training, thermal biofeedback combined with relaxation training, electromyographic biofeedback, and cognitive-behavioral therapy may be considered as treatment options for prevention of migraine (Grade A). Specific recommendations regarding which of these to use for specific patients cannot be made.
- Behavioral therapy may be combined with preventive drug therapy to achieve additional clinical improvement for migraine relief (Grade B).
- Evidence-based treatment recommendations regarding the use of hypnosis, acupuncture, transcutaneous electrical nerve stimulation, chiropractic or osteopathic cervical manipulation, occlusal adjustment, and hyperbaric oxygen as preventive or acute therapy for migraine are not yet possible.

Many migraine patients try nonpharmacologic treatment to manage their headaches *before* they begin drug therapy or concurrently *with* drug therapy. Behavioral treatments are classified into three broad categories: relaxation training, biofeedback therapy, and cognitive-behavioral (stress-management) training. Physical treatment includes acupuncture, cervical manipulation, and mobilization therapy. These are treatment options for headache sufferers who have one or more of the following characteristics:

- Preference for nonpharmacologic interventions
- Poor tolerance to specific pharmacologic treatments
- Medical contraindications to specific pharmacologic treatments
- Insufficient or no response to pharmacologic treatment
- Pregnancy, planned pregnancy, or nursing
- History of long-term, frequent, or excessive use of analgesic or acute medications that can aggravate headache problems (or lead to decreased responsiveness to other pharmacotherapies)
- Significant stress or deficient stress-coping skills

REFERENCES

Andrasik F, Buse DC, Grazzi L. Behavioral medicine for migraine and medication overuse headache. *Curr Pain Headache Rep*. 2009;13(3):241–248.

Busch V, Gaul C. Exercise in migraine therapy—is there any evidence for efficacy? A critical review. *Headache*. 2008;48(6):890–899.

Nestoriuc Y, Martin A, Rief W, Andrasik F. Biofeedback treatment for headache disorders: a comprehensive efficacy review. *Appl Psychophysiol Biofeedback*. 2008;33(3):125–140.

Silberstein SD, Edlund W. Practice parameter: evidence-based guidelines for migraine headache (an evidence-based review): report of the quality standards subcommittee of the American academy of neurology. *Neurology*. 2000;55(6):754–762.

Wöber C, Brannath W, Schmidt K, et al. Prospective analysis of factors related to migraine attacks: the PAMINA study. *Cephalalgia*. 2007:27(4):304–314.

12 Headache in the Emergency Department

INTRODUCTION

Patients who present to the emergency department (ED) with a chief complaint of headache often have severe or disabling migraine. These patients often have had a primary headache disorder with an insufficient overall management plan. However, unusual primary headaches and secondary causes must always be considered when a patient presents emergently.

It is important to assess for red flags (i.e., using the SNOOP mnemonic, see Chapter 3) indicating a potential secondary cause for the headache, even if clinical features conform well to the diagnostic criteria for a primary headache disorder. Subarachnoid hemorrhage may mimic migraine and can improve with migraine-specific treatment. Treatment response before the diagnostic evaluation is completed gives a false sense of security and can lead to disastrous outcomes if the patient has improved and the underlying cause has not been addressed. Look for sudden (thunderclap) onset headache; if absent, nuchal rigidity may be present. Pay particular attention to the following in the physical examination:

- Vital signs: fever, hypertension, hypotension
- Carotid and vertebral arteries: palpate for tenderness, auscultate for bruits
- Temporal arteries: palpate for tenderness and pulsatility
- Neurologic examination
  - Mental status: level of consciousness, presence of delusions or hallucinations
  - Fundi, pupils: papilledema, retinal hemorrhage, pupillary asymmetry and reactivity
  - Eyes: diplopia, dysconjugate gaze, injection, visual field deficit
  - Neck: differentiate stiffness from muscle spasm and meningeal irritation
  - Extremities: focal weakness or sensory loss, limb ataxia, asymmetric reflexes, Babinski sign
  - Gait and station: ataxia, hemiparesis, Romberg sign

DIAGNOSTIC APPROACH

Uncomplicated migraine with a history and examination that contain no red flags requires no diagnostic testing, and it is most appropriate simply to treat.

TABLE 12.1 Strongest Predictors of Migraine Diagnosis

- Nausea
  - Are you nauseated or sick to your stomach when you have a headache?
- Disability
  - Has a headache limited your activities for a day or more in the last 3 months?
- Photophobia
  - Does light bother you when you have a headache?
    2 out of 3 symptoms: 93%
    3 out of 3 symptoms: 98%

Assessment

Does the patient have migraine? A simple three-question inventory called ID Migraine ™ serves as a moderately sensitive (81%) and specific (75%) screening tool with excellent positive predictive value (93%) for the presence of migraine (Table 12.1).

A patient in the ED probably already fulfills the second question (disability), so simply asking about nausea and photosensitivity should point in the direction of migraine. Patients presenting to the ED with severe nonmigrainous headache may be suffering from cluster headache; consider this if photophobia and nausea are absent. However, some patients with cluster headache also experience migrainous features. Because cluster attacks typically do not last more than 3 hours, most will not come to evaluation before the attack is over.

Should treatment fail, the accuracy of the diagnosis may be called into question and a more detailed diagnostic evaluation is undertaken. Revisit the history to ensure that the primary diagnosis is correct and no red flags have been missed. If the diagnosis seems correct and no other red flags exist, alternative treatments should be tried. Failure to respond to treatment, however, may be considered a red flag in and of itself.

Systemic Symptoms (Fever, Weight Loss), Secondary Risks (HIV, Immunosuppression, Known Cancer)

These may indicate a serious underlying medical illness such as widespread infection that could penetrate the central nervous system (CNS) and lead to headache, or in the case of HIV, make one susceptible to CNS infection. Although evidence suggests that most headaches are not caused or worsened by primary and metastatic brain tumors, headache is the presenting symptom in up to 20% of cases and develops eventually in 60%. Migraineurs may be more susceptible to brain tumor headache.

Neurologic Symptoms/Signs (Altered Consciousness, Focal Deficits)

When present, intracranial pathology such as stroke must be ruled out. CT scan is the best first test because it is obtained quickly and will reveal most acute processes in the cranial vault. When CT is negative or inconclusive, MRI should be obtained. Gadolinium is helpful in assessing for tumors, acute demyelination, and low cerebrospinal fluid (CSF) pressure/volume (pachymeningeal enhancement occurs). Magnetic resonance angiography (MRA) will reveal medium- to large-sized aneurysms and arterial dissections. Magnetic resonance venography (MRV) will reveal venous sinus thrombosis or stenosis. When MRI is contraindicated, CT with contrast, CTA, and CTV can be used.

Onset—Sudden or Split-Second

"Thunderclap headache" can be benign, but several secondary causes must be ruled out. The differential diagnosis includes subarachnoid hemorrhage, unruptured intracranial aneurysm, aneurysmal expansion or thrombosis, cervical arterial dissection, cerebral venous thrombosis, retroclival hematoma, pituitary apoplexy, stroke, reversible cerebral vasoconstriction syndrome, spontaneous CSF leak, hypertensive crisis, intracranial infection, and colloid cyst of the third ventricle. CT, lumbar puncture, and MRI (including arteriography and venography) will exclude or confirm these causes in the vast majority of cases.

Older—New or Progressive Over Age 50

Migraine prevalence peaks in middle age, but incidence typically is not after age 50. Giant cell arteritis is a disorder of elderly individuals presenting with new or progressive headache that may be indistinguishable from typical primary headaches. Often, but not always, a tender, firm, pulseless temporal artery, jaw claudication, constitutional signs, and visual symptoms are present. Prompt recognition and treatment are vital in preventing permanent neurological sequelae, most notably blindness and stroke.

Prior History—First, Newly Progressive, or Different from the Patient's Usual Headaches

Any unusual headache beyond what is described earlier deserves further investigation.

Dutto et al. have reported an efficient means of triaging nontraumatic headache cases in the ED. They divided patients into three subgroups that reflect the essentials of the SNOOP mnemonic. The first subgroup included patients with severe headache (worst-ever headache);

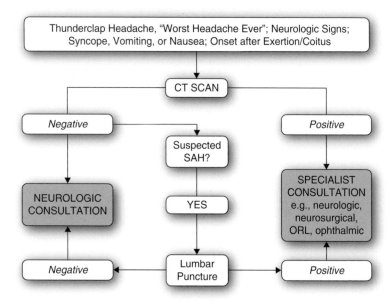

FIGURE 12.1 First subgroup. ORL, otorhinolaryngologic; SAH, subarachnoid hemorrhage.

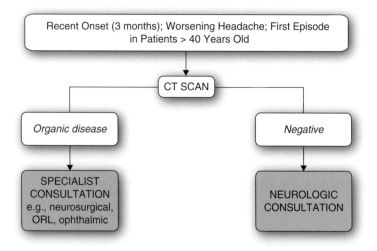

FIGURE 12.2 Second subgroup. ORL, otorhinolaryngologic.

thunderclap headache; headache accompanied by clinical findings (focal or general); headache with vomiting or syncope at onset; and headaches following exertion or sexual intercourse (Figure 12.1; see Chapter 3 for more details).

The second subgroup included patients with headache of recent onset (weeks or months); worsening or persistent headache; and people more than age 40 describing their first headache episode (Figure 12.2).

The third subgroup included patients with a known history of headache who suffered an attack that was very similar in type to those in the past, but differed in terms of length, intensity, or resistance to usual analgesic therapy (Figure 12.3).

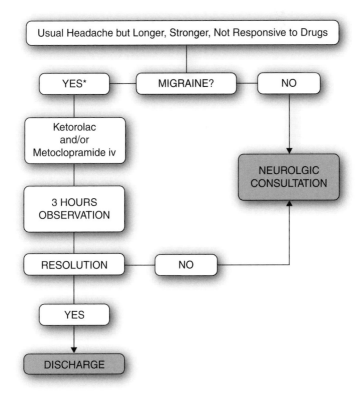

FIGURE 12.3 Third subgroup.
Source: Dutto L, Meineri P, Melchio R, Bracco C, Lauria G, Sciolla A, Pomero F, Sturlese U, Grasso E, Tartaglino B. Nontraumatic headaches in the ER: Evaluation of a clinical pathway. Headache 2009;49;1174-1185

TREATMENTS

For migraine, a combination of medications from various classes or repeating doses after 2 hours might be necessary to abort the headache. See Table 12.2 for some examples of intravenous medications (Chapter 13). Use oxygen or subcutaneous sumatriptan for acute cluster headache (Chapter 14). For secondary headaches, address the underlying cause and treat the headache symptomatically. In almost all cases of primary headache, *opioids must be avoided!* Exceptions may include pregnancy, trauma, and unusual headache syndromes. Most primary headache disorders are made worse by opioid exposure. Moreover, animal experimentation has shown that rats administered opioids have a preference for the place in their environment at which the opioids were administered; if this translates to humans, it would make return visits to the ED more likely when opioids are used to treat headache.

TABLE 12.2 Migraine Terminators

A. *NSAIDs and corticosteroids*—nonspecific analgesics, caution advised in those with hepatic or renal impairment, diabetes, or gastritis. Choose one of the following drugs:
   a. Ketorolac (Toradol) 30 mg IV
   b. Methylprednisolone (Solu-Medrol) 100 to 200 mg
   c. Dexamethasone (Decadron) 10 to 40 mg
B. *Neuroleptics*—used alone and as pretreatment to DHE to offset nausea; diphenhydramine (Benadryl) 25 to 50 mg, lorazepam (Ativan) 0.5 to 1 mg, and/or benztropine (Cogentin) 1 mg often given before neuroleptic to mitigate akathisia; must check EKG and avoid if QTc > 460 for women or > 450 for men (except metoclopramide, which does not prolong QTc)
   a. Metoclopramide (Reglan) 10 to 20 mg IV
   b. Prochlorperazine (Compazine) 10 to 20 mg IV, IM
   c. Droperidol (Inapsine) 0.625 to 2.5 mg IV or IM
   d. Chlorpromazine (Thorazine) 12.5 to 100 mg po, IV (up to 50 mg only; do not give IM—too painful)
   e. Haloperidol (Haldol) 1 to 10 mg IV
C. *DHE* 0.5 to 1 mg IV push—migraine-specific but also helpful in cluster; must not be administered if a triptan was taken in the preceding 24 hours; contraindicated in patients with history of, or at high risk for, MI or stroke
D. *Anticonvulsants*—given as rapid infusions (over 10 to 20 minutes) can be useful
   a. *Valproic acid*—500 to 1000 mg, can also be useful for cluster headache
   b. *Levetiracetam*—1000 to 2000 mg, maximum recommended dose is 3000 mg/day (although higher doses have been used)
E. *Magnesium sulfate*—1 to 2 g IVPB (tends to burn and caustic to veins)

Abbreviations: DHE, dihyroergotamine; NSAIDs, nonsteroidal anti-inflammatory drugs.

REFERENCES

Dutto L, Meineri P, Melchio R, et al. Nontraumatic headaches in the emergency department: evaluation of a clinical pathway. *Headache*. 2009;49(8):1174–1185.

Kelly AM. Migraine: pharmacotherapy in the emergency department. *J Accid Emerg Med*. 2000;17(4):241–245.

Lipton RB, Dodick D, Sadovsky R, et al. A self-administered screener for migraine in primary care: the ID migraine™ validation study. *Neurology*. 2003;61(3):375–382.

Schankin CJ, Ferrari U, Reinisch VM, Birnbaum T, Goldbrunner R, Straube A. Characteristics of brain tumour-associated headache. *Cephalalgia*. 2007;27(8):904–911.

Schwedt TJ, Matharu MS, Dodick DW. Thunderclap headache. *Lancet Neurol*. 2006;5(7):621–631.

13 Infusion and Inpatient Treatment

Headache varies from mild to severely disabling. At one extreme is a subgroup of patients whose headaches are so severe and debilitating that they cannot be treated as outpatients and need to be hospitalized. Inpatient treatment programs are available in most countries that have headache experts. Those who do not have a formal treatment program almost certainly have nonprogramatic hospitalizations to treat primary headache (Table 13.1).

Patients are hospitalized for a number of reasons. These include:

- Migraine status: episodic migraine lasting longer than 3 days and refractory to multiple outpatient treatments, including emergency room or infusion treatments
- Chronic daily headache (transformed migraine, chronic tension-type headache, new daily persistent headache, or hemicrania continua) or posttraumatic headache, with either:
  - Severe disability (i.e., inability to work, severe absenteeism) and have failed multiple outpatient treatments and at least 2 days of infusion center treatment

TABLE 13.1 International Headache Society Members with Inpatient Headache Programs

Admit			Do Not Admit
Argentina	France	Poland	Canada
Australia	Germany	Romania	Turkey
Austria	Greece	Russia	Jordan
Belgium	Hungary	Slovakia	Portugal
Bosnia	India	Spain	
Brazil	Israel	Sweden	
Bulgaria	Italy	Taiwan	
China	Japan	Ukraine	
Croatia	Kazakhstan	United Kingdom	
Czech Republic	Latvia	United States	
Denmark	Philippines		

Source: Modified from The International Headache Society and The European Headache Federation, 1995.

- Medication overuse for which outpatient treatment is too risky or unlikely to succeed
- Psychiatric or medical disease that makes outpatient management risky or unlikely to succeed
■ Intractable cluster headaches
■ Prolonged migraine aura refractory to outpatient measures
■ Secondary headache with the possibility of brain injury (e.g., thunderclap headache because of dissection)
■ Diagnostic mysteries or uncertainties and concern for ominous cause of headache

Since inpatient treatment is often used for patients who are overusing analgesics (or are at high risk for analgesic overuse), inpatients should not be given analgesics other than nonsteroidal anti-inflammatory drugs (NSAIDs). They should not receive opioids, barbiturates, or even acetaminophen. Giving these drugs sends the wrong message; patients are in the hospital to avoid acute medication overuse. This subgroup of patients already suffers from daily headaches and usually have analgesic overuse, and the medication may lead to other treatments (such as intravenous [IV] dihydroergotamine [DHE]) becoming ineffective.

In our program, the typical inpatient receives:

■ IV neuroleptics/nausea medicines (often metoclopramide), followed by IV DHE every 8 hours
■ prn medication with some sedative properties (i.e., po chlorpromazine, IV droperidol, or po olanzapine) that may be given between doses of DHE for a severe headache
■ A regimen to avoid physical withdrawal to opioids or barbiturates (methadone, clonidine, or phenobarbital)

If the patient's headache does not respond after several days, the regimen is augmented (i.e., IV steroids added) or changed (IV lidocaine if DHE is contraindicated or patient has failed IV DHE in the past, or if it seems a long length of stay will be required).

The goal of hospitalization is for the patient to be headache-free or have minimal headache (i.e., 1/10) on discharge. For some, the goal is to alter the headache profile and pain behaviors, allowing successful outpatient therapy. Hospitalization can dramatically improve a patient's life and get them on the path to recovery.

In centers that do not offer infusion center treatment, the average hospitalization is about 3 days. (Most patients become completely headache-free on the third or fourth day and are discharged 24 hours later.) Duration is 7 to 21 days at regional headache centers that treat the most refractory patients. One constraint on length of stay is the safety of repetitive IV DHE: safety beyond 7 days (21 mg; 3 mg/day × 7 days) has not been established. Furthermore, the likelihood of the patient becoming headache-free diminishes after day 5 or 6. With the increasing use of IV lidocaine, prolonged hospitalization (>8 days) is becoming more common, as many patients take several days to begin to respond to this treatment.

Unless it is contraindicated or the patient was overusing DHE prior to hospitalization, most of our patients receive DHE. Contraindications include coronary artery disease, peripheral vascular disease, poorly controlled hypertension, large or medium vessel stroke, and prolonged aura or basilar migraine. Patients who receive DHE in the hospital should have an electrocardiogram (EKG) prior to beginning treatment. If a patient does not respond after 48 hours, the regimen is usually changed or augmented by the addition of methylprednisolone, ketorolac, or IV valproic acid. Other strategies include around-the-clock dosing of olanzapine, IV push of chlorpromazine, or increasing the potency or dose of the neuroleptic/antinausea medicine.

All inpatients with chronic daily headache or posttraumatic headache are seen in consultation by our psychiatry and psychology services. The consultants provide us with a 5 Axis DSM IV diagnosis, an outpatient behavioral management plan appropriate for the patient, and psychopharmacologic advice. Only rarely will the psychologist and psychiatrist not be consulted (e.g., secondary headache or episodic cluster).

Less extreme are patients who can be managed in an infusion center. Infusion center treatment is typically given when the following conditions exist:

- Migraine status with inability to work or go to school, refractory to one or more rescue treatments at home
- Chronic daily headache with significant disability
- Medication overuse headache of simple analgesics or small doses of butalbital, triptans, or opioids
- Prolonged aura without motor symptoms not progressively worsening

The goals of infusion center treatment are similar to those of hospitalization. Many different medications are used (Table 13.2), but the medicine is concentrated within a shorter period of time (i.e., 2 mg of DHE within 3 hours, 7.5 mg of droperidol within 4 hours) and the patient may have more side effects as a tradeoff for faster relief. Patients are not allowed to drive

TABLE 13.2 Treatments used at Jefferson Headache Center for the Inpatient and Infusion Center Management of Severe Headache

---

Major Classes And Drugs

- Neuroleptics
  - Haloperidol
  - Chlorpromazine
  - Droperidol
  - Prochlorperazine
  - Olanzapine
  - Metoclopramide
  - Promethazine
- Dihydroergotamine
- Steroids
- Nonsteroidal anti-inflammatory drugs
- Magnesium sulfate
- Valproic acid
- Levetiracetam
- Lidocaine
- Local anesthetics for nerve block and/or trigger point injection
- Adjuncts (little headache effect)
  - Ondansetron
  - Lorazepam
  - Benzotropine
  - Diphenhydramine
  - Clonidine
  - Phenobarbital
  - Atropine diphenoxylate

---

following infusion center treatment, and we advise that a friend or relative drive the patient home, although public transportation may be appropriate if less sedating medications are used or the patient is kept an extra hour to allow recuperation from the sedation. Patients may be admitted to the hospital from the infusion center if their pain is so severe that discharge to home is inadvisable. Rarely, a patient will need to be hospitalized from the infusion center because of side effects.

The art of inpatient management is to find the most effective treatment possible, thus shortening length of stay while managing risk and not causing unmanageable or unacceptable side effects. Since IV neuroleptics are the backbone of an inpatient treatment regimen, we have made the following observations:

Neuroleptics

1. **Efficacy**: for headache pain

<u>Maximum 24-hour dose</u>
(in headache center)

More Effective

Less Effective

- ▶ IV haloperidol
  (1–5 mg q 6–8 hours)   100 mg
- ▶ IVP chlorpromazine
  (12.5 to 50 mg q 6–8 hours)   50 mg
- ▶ IV droperidol
  (0.625 to 2.5 mg q 6–8 hours)   10 mg
- ▶ IV prochlorperazine
  (5–10 mg q 6–8 hours)   40 mg
- ▶ IV drip chlorpromazine
  (12.5 to 50 mg q 6–8 hours)   400 mg
- ▶ po olanzapine
  (5–10 prn, max 20 mg in 24 hours) 20 mg
- ▶ po chlorpromazine (25–50 mg)   400 mg
- ▶ IV metoclopramide (10 mg)   60 mg
- ▶ IV promethazine (12.5–50 mg) 100 mg

{only give IV w/PICC line otherwise po/pr due to risk of phlebitis; tissue drainage if infiltrated}

2. **Side effects**:

a) *Sedation*

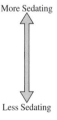

More Sedating

Less Sedating

- ▶ IV chlorpromazine
- ▶ IV droperidol
- ▶ IV promethazine
- ▶ po chlorpromazine
- ▶ IV haloperidol
- ▶ IV prochlorperazine
- ▶ po olanzapine
- ▶ po metoclopramide

b) *Dystonia/Akathisia* Dystonia is involuntary sustained contraction of a group of muscles causing movement of a joint. Akathisia is a feeling of inner restlessness associated with a desire to move. These are among the most common side effects.

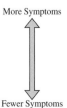

More Symptoms

Fewer Symptoms

- ▶ Haloperidol
- ▶ Droperidol
- ▶ Prochlorperazine
- ▶ Metoclopramide
- ▶ Chlorpromazine
- ▶ Promethazine
- ▶ Olanzapine

Patients coming off opioids sometimes experience restlessness and an urge to move. The differential includes undiagnosed restless legs syndrome (RLS). Nocturnal symptoms and relief by walking differentiate RLS from akathisia. Dopamine blockers generally worsen it. Rather than stopping the neuroleptic and having an unsuccessful hospitalization, we add gabapentin or clonazepam at bedtime. If a patient is on a dopamine agonist for RLS, we usually switch to clonazepam during the hospitalization.

c) *Anticholinergic*

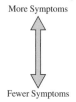
More Symptoms / Fewer Symptoms

▶ Chlorpromazine
▶ Promethazine
▶ Prochlorperazine
▶ Droperidol
▶ Metoclopramide
▶ Olanzapine

An important consideration during hospitalization is the risk of prolonging the QTc beyond 500 ms, potentially leading to Torsades de pointes, a potentially fatal cardiac arrhythmia caused by various medications commonly used for hospitalized headache patients. We do daily EKGs to identify QTc prolongation. If QTc prolongation occurs, we adjust the dose.

■ *Prolonged QT*: droperidol >> chlorpromazine + prochlorperazine > others; olanzapine doubtful; metoclopramide none. Patients receiving neuroleptics other than metoclopramide get EKG before the first dose and daily thereafter. Mg, Ca, and K should be checked (K to be > 4.0). QTc above 450 is "gray zone" (stop or reduce dose) and QTc above 500 is "red zone" (absolute contraindication). Bradycardia, abnormal EKG, hypomagnesemia, hypokalemia, and change in QTc of more than 60 ms are other risk factors for Torsades de pointes associated with prolonged QT syndrome.

■ Other medications that can cause QT prolongation include:
  • Methadone
  • Clarithromycin
  • Erythromycin
  • Venlafaxine
  • Tizanidine
  • Azithromycin
  • Levofloxacin
  • Lithium
  • Ondansetron

■ *Risk of tardive akathisia*: theoretically haloperidol > droperidol > prochlorperazine > metoclopramide > chlorpromazine > promethazine > olanzapine

DHE is a 5-HT1 agonist (hence antimigraine); dopamine agonist (hence pronausea); and α-adrenergic blocker. The inpatient dose is 0.2 to 1.0 mg IV every 8 hours (generally 0.5 mg first, repeated in 1 hour if tolerated, then raised thereafter) maximum of 3 mg a day; limit 7 consecutive days in hospital. In the infusion center, one may repeat DHE and give up to 2 mg in 2 to 3 hours. DHE is a vasoconstrictor (veins>>arteries) and should be given cautiously in the presence of Raynaud's disease. Assess cardiac and stroke risk. Chest symptoms are so common that diagnostic testing is usually not warranted unless angina is suspected. There may be a flushing reaction—warmth or pressure in the neck, chest, face, or sometimes entire trunk—following DHE administration. It is most intense the first time the patient is exposed to a given dose. This side effect is not a contraindication for ongoing use and decreases with subsequent doses (IV>>IM>>IN). Nausea often occurs the first time a patient is given DHE but decreases over subsequent doses (IV>>IM>>IN). Diarrhea may occur, usually after a few days (in infusion center can space 3 hours apart to minimize). Aching or sore legs can also occur.

Corticosteroids. We generally use IV methylprednisolone 100 to 200 mg every 12 hours for up to 3 days. We check glucose twice a day and cover with sliding scale insulin. Gastrointestinal bleeding is a major concern with steroid use; therefore, we give gastrointestinal protection (H2 blocker or PPI). Activation of mania or other psychiatric symptoms occurs infrequently. We use the psychiatric consultation to identify individuals at risk for this complication.

Nonsteroidal anti-inflammatory drugs. There is a high risk of gastrointestinal bleeding or renal injury if NSAIDs are used too long. We limit ketorolac to 30 mg IV for a maximum of 3 consecutive days. We do not use corticosteroids concurrently and we give gastrointestinal protection.

Magnesium sulfate is probably safe but its benefit is small. It tends to sclerose veins, so it is better to give it only if the patient has a PICC line or will be discharged soon. We give 1 g IV every 8 to 24 hours in the hospital. It is contraindicated in the presence of renal insufficiency. Monitor reflexes daily (when they disappear, the patient has had too much) and measure levels after 3 days. Allow 1.5 times top normal magnesium level if no side effects occur.

IV valproic acid has been studied open label and may be effective in single or repetitive doses. We generally give 250 to 500 mg IVP (one time dose, occasionally may repeat; recently published dosing schedule every 8 hours). May give 500 to 1000 mg IV **rapid infusion** (adjust rate to infuse over 10 minutes). Watch for tremor, encephalopathy, and nausea with prolonged use; stop medication and consider checking ammonia level. We have found that IV lidocaine increases the risk of reversible encephalopathy, so we avoid this combination.

IV levetiracetam. One poster has suggested that IV levetiracetam is effective for severe migraine. The dose is 1000 mg (in one case series 2000 mg was used as a one-time dose). There are few side effects. One concern is the possibility of rare dysphoria/mood changes.

IV lidocaine has been studied in several case series and appears to be effective. We initiate telemetry monitoring, check EKG, magnesium, and potassium before starting the drug, then daily EKG and labs every 2 to 4 days, or as needed. Start lidocaine 1 mg/minute × 4 hours then **automatically increase** to 2 mg/minute. Check the lidocaine level the next morning, then after any dose change or if indicated by the clinical situation. In our experience, the patient responds better when lidocaine levels are near the top of the "therapeutic range," about 4 to 5.

Side effects are common and principally involve the central nervous system, including blurry vision, tremor, vivid dreams, hallucinations, and psychosis. Tachycardia may occur but generally does not lead to discontinuation.

Local anesthetics (for nerve block and or trigger point injection)

Greater occipital nerve blocks are effective in migraine, cluster headache (with corticosteroids), and posttraumatic headache. Paraspinal muscle injections were effective in another study. Once a patient begins to improve, occipital nerve block is a useful adjuvant.

ADVERSE EVENTS

Some adverse events need urgent management. Encephalopathies may be due to valproate or lidocaine. Excessive sedation is treated by reducing the dose of sedating medication or switching to another one. Anticholinergic toxicity can present with a Korsakov amnesic syndrome. This can be aggravated by lorazepam or valproic acid, but reverses quickly.

Serotonin syndrome may present with alterations in mental status, behavior, autonomic nervous system function, and neuromuscular activity. Altered neuromuscular function is the most commonly reported symptom, presenting as myoclonus, hyperreflexia with clonus, and/or muscle rigidity, in particular, bilateral lower extremity rigidity. Changes in cognition and behavior, such as confusion or agitation, are common, but may be undetected or dismissed as a manifestation of an underlying psychiatric condition. Diaphoresis, hyperthermia, hypertension, and tachycardia are the most prevalent reported autonomic nervous system symptoms.

Neuroleptic malignant syndrome can be a diagnostic challenge. Compared with serotonin syndrome, neuroleptic malignant syndrome patients are more toxic with greater impairment of consciousness, more hyperthermia (with higher temperatures), lead-pipe muscle rigidity, and lack of myoclonus. Patients with neuroleptic malignant syndrome are more likely to have metabolic acidosis and elevations in liver function tests, white blood cell count, and creatine kinase.

ADJUNCTS

Table 13.3 demonstrates commonly used adjuncts during hospitalization.

TABLE 13.3 Adjunctive Medications Used in Infusion Center and Hospital

Medication	Purpose	Dosage
Ondansetron	Antinauseant without risk of extrapyramidal side effects	4 to 8 mg IV q 8 hours
Lorazepam	Sedation or antianxiety	0.5 to 1 mg IV q 6 hours or 0.5 to 2 mg po q 6 hours
Benztropine	Anticholinergic to treat extrapyramidal side effects	0.5 to 1 mg po/IM q 8 hours
Diphenhydramine	Anticholinergic to treat extrapyramidal side effects	50 mg IV q 4 hours
Methadone	Treat opioid withdrawal	2.5 to 10 mg po daily-tid[a]
Phenobarbital	Treat barbiturate/butalbital withdrawal	100 mg IM/IV then 100 mg IM/IV q 12 hours prn or 30 to 60 mg po qhs for up to 5 days
Clonidine	Treat opioid withdrawal	0.1 to 0.2 mg bid/tid
Atropine diphenoxylate	Diarrhea due to DHE	1 to 2 tablets prn (no maximum) diarrhea

[a] Titrate to mild to moderate opioid withdrawal symptoms. Do not give equianalgesic doses—this is too much. We suggest using a conversion calculator with dose reduction of 50% to account for incomplete cross-tolerance. Many calculators are freely available. Here is a link to one: http://www.globalrph.com/narcoticonv.htm

REFERENCES

Freitag FG, Lake III A, Lipton RB, Cady, R, for the United States Headache Guidelines Consortium, Section on Inpatient Treatment. Inpatient treatment of headache: an evidence-based assessment. *Headache.* 2004;44:342–360.

Kabbouche MA, Powers SW, Segers A, et al. Inpatient treatment of status migraine with dihydroergotamine in children and adolescents. *Headache.* 2009;49:106–109.

Relja G, Granato A, Bratina A, Antonello RM, Zorzon M. Outcome of medication headache after abrupt inpatient withdrawal. *Cephalalgia.* 2006;26:589–595.

The International Headache Society and The European Headache Federation, eds. *Headache Research Worldwide: Headache Centers Directory.* München, Germany: Arcis-Verlag; 1995.

Williams DR, Stark RJ. Intravenous lignocaine (lidocaine) infusion for the treatment of chronic daily headache with substantial medication overuse. *Cephalalgia.* 2003;23:963–971.

SAMPLE ADMISSION ORDERS

ADMIT TO: Headache Unit

ATTENDING: _____ FELLOW: _____ RESIDENT: _____ BEEPER: _____

Diagnosis

- ☐ Transformed migraine
- ☐ Migraine status
- ☐ Medication overuse headache
  - ☐ Analgesics ☐ Opioids ☐ triptans ☐ butalbital ☐ mixed
- ☐ Cluster headache
- ☐ New daily persistent headache

- ☐ Hemicrania Continua
- ☐ Post traumatic headache
- ☐ Idiopathic intracranial hypertension
- ☐ Low pressure/volume headache
- ☐ Other:

Allergies

_____ ☐ No Known Allergies   ☐ Latex Allergy

☐ Other _____

Admission Orders

- ☐ Baseline ECG, physician/NP to check prior to administration of initial medications
- ☐ Baseline vital signs and neuro check
- ☐ Peripheral IV insertion
- ☐ PICC insertion - double lumen

IV Fluids

☐ 0.9 NSS   ☐ D5W/0.45 NSS   ☐ Other:

Rate _____ ml/hour x _____ liters

Routine Orders

- ☐ Telemetry, vital sign Q 4 hours review telemetry strips Q 8 hours and document measurements. Notify resident if QTc > 450 (men) or >460 (women)
- ☐ Vital Signs Q 8 hours
- ☐ Neuro checks Q _____ hours
- ☐ I/O Q shift
- ☐ Accuchecks and sliding scale insulin BID
- ☐ ECG daily
- ☐ Other _____

Diet

- ☐ House
- ☐ Low Caffeine
- ☐ 1800 ADA diet
- ☐ Cardiac Prudent diet
- ☐ Other _____

Activity

- ☐ OOB ad lib
- ☐ OOB assist
- ☐ Sequential compression boots while in bed

Date: _____ Time: _____ **Physician Signnature:** _____

Admission Labs

- [ ] CBC with diff
- [ ] Basic Metabolic Panel
- [ ] Comprehensive Metabolic Panel
- [ ] Ionized Calcium
- [ ] Magnesium
- [ ] Phosphate
- [ ] PT/PTT
- [ ] Beta Test
- [ ] Drug levels:

- [ ] TSH
- [ ] ESR
- [ ] RPR
- [ ] ANA and Panel if positive
- [ ] Urine drug screen [ ] 6 [ ] 9
- [ ] U/A
- [ ] Urine Culture
- [ ] Other:

Other Tests

- [ ] MRI brain [ ] with gadolinium [ ] with gadolinium indication:
- [ ] MRI C-Spine [ ] with gadolinium [ ] with gadolinium indication:
- [ ] MRA [ ] brain [ ] neck indication:
- [ ] MRV brain indication:
- [ ] Chest x-ray PA/lateral indication:
- [ ] Nuclear Cistemogram indication:
- [ ] CT myelogram indication:
- [ ] Other _____

Consults

- [ ] Hospitalist
- [ ] Psychiatry
- [ ] Neuropsychology
- [ ] Social Services regarding:
- [ ] Dietician/Nutritionist
- [ ] Physical Therapy for evaluation and treatment of:
- [ ] Other _____

Pre-Medication

- [ ] None
- [ ] Diphenhydramine (Benadryl) _____ mg IV
    - [ ] Q ___ hours prior to anti-emetic
    - OR [ ] timed: _____

- [ ] Lorazepam (Ativan) _____ mg IV
    - [ ] Q ___ hours
    - OR [ ] timed: _____

- [ ] Benztropine (Cogentin) 1mg IM
    - [ ] Q ___ hours
    - OR [ ] timed: _____

- [ ] Other _____

Date: Time: Physician Signnature:

Anti-Emotics

☐ Metodopramide (Reglan) _____ mg IV

☐ Q ___ hours

OR ☐ timed: _____

☐ Prochlorperazine (Compazine) _____ mg IV

☐ Q ___ hours

OR ☐ timed: _____

☐ Droperidol (Inapsine) _____ mg IV

☐ Q ___ hours

OR ☐ timed: _____

☐ Promethazine (Phenergan) _____ mg IV

☐ Q ___ hours

OR ☐ timed: _____

☐ Chlorpromazine (Thorazine) _____ mg IV

☐ 25mg in 100mL NSS over 30 minutes

☐ 50mg in 100mL NSS over 30 minutes

☐ Q ___ hours

OR ☐ timed: _____

☐ Haloperidol (Haldol) _____ mg IV

☐ Q ___ hours

OR ☐ timed: _____

☐ Ondansetron (Zofran) _____ mg IV

☐ Q ___ hours

OR ☐ timed: _____

Pain Medications

☐ Dihydroergotamine (DHE) _____ mg IVP after anti-emetic

over 3 minutes then check pulse and BP 5, 15 and 30 minutes after administration of first 2 doses
Repeat in one hour if headache not relieved then:

☐ Q ___ hours

OR ☐ timed: _____

HOLD DHE AND NOTIFY MD IF:

-Baseline SBP > 150 or DBP > 95

-SBP increases or decreases by > 30mm Hg

-DBP increases or decreases by > 15mm Hg

Patient develops chest pain, changes in mental status, or severe nausea

Date: **Time:**   **Physician Signature:**

Pain Medications (cont'd)

☐ Lidocaine (standard concentration in 2 grams in 250mL D5W) 1mg/min IV (7.5 mL.hour) X 4 hours then increase to 2mg/min IV (15 mL/hour)

☐ Lidocaine _____ mg/min IV

☐ Ketorolac (Toradol) 30mg IVP

    ☐ Q _____ hours x 3 days

OR ☐ timed: _____

☐ Magnesium 1 gram in 100mL D5W over 30 minutes

☐ Magnesium 2 grams in 200mL D5W over 60 minutes

    ☐ Q _____ hours

OR ☐ timed: _____

☐ Valproic Acid (Depacon)

    ☐ 500mg in 100 mL NSS over 20 minutes

    ☐ 1 gram in 100 mL NSS over 20 minutes

    ☐ Q _____ hours

OR ☐ timed: _____

☐ Methylprednisolone (Solu-Medrol) 125mg IV in 100mL D5W over 30 minutes x 6 doses

    ☐ Q _____ hours

OR ☐ timed: _____

☐ Caffeine 500 mg IV in 50 mL D5W over 20 minutes BID at 7AM and 1PM

☐ Other _____

Other Medications

☐ Methadone (Dolophine) _____ mg PO on arrival

    Day 1: _____

    Day 2: _____

    Day 3: _____

    and _____ mg PO Q _____ hours PRN withdrawal symptoms not relieved by Clonidine or Lorazepam

☐ Phenobarbital _____ mg   ☐ IM ☐ IV ☐ PO on arrival

    Day 1: _____ mg PO HS

    Day 2: _____ mg PO HS

    Day 3: _____ mg PO HS

    and _____ mg   ☐ IM ☐ IV ☐ PO Q _____ hours PRN withdrawal symptoms

☐ Clonidine _____ mg ☐ PO Q _____ hours ☐ Patch Q 7 days ☐ Q _____ PRN withdrawal symptoms

☐ Other _____

Date: **Time:**   **Physician Signature:**

For Severe Breakthrough Pain

☐ Olanzapine (Zyprexa) _____ mg PO Q _____ hours PRN

☐ Ketorolac (Toradol) _____ mg IVP Q _____ hours PRN

☐ Naproxen 500 mg PO Q _____ hours PRN

☐ Other: _____

Other PRN Medications

☐ Zolpidem (Ambien)_____ mg PO QHS PRN sleep

☐ Senna (Senokot) one tablet PO BID PRN constipation

☐ Docusate Sodium (Colace) 100 mg PO BIO PRN constipation

☐ Bisacodyl (Dulcolax) _____ mg ☐ PO ☐ PR daily PRN for constipation

☐ Diphenoxylate/Atropine (Lomotil) one tablet PO PRN after each loose stool (Limit of 5 doses/day)

☐ Diphenhydramine (Benadryl) _____ mg IVPB Q 6 hours PRN dystonic reaction, akethesia, itch

☐ Lorazepam (Ativan) _____ mg ☐ IV ☐ PO Q _____ hours PRN akethesia, anxiety, withdrawal

☐ Benztropine (cogentin) 1mg IM Q 6 hours PRN severe dystonic reaction

☐ Other _____

Other Medications

_____

_____

_____

_____

_____

_____

_____

_____

_____

Date: Time: Physician Signature:

14 Cluster Headache

Cluster headache (CH) is a primary headache disorder characterized by a unilateral headache with autonomic features. The headache lasts 15 to 180 minutes. CH is the most common trigeminal autonomic cephalgia (TAC) and may have a prevalence of up to 2 per 1000 persons.

The International Classification of Headache Disorders II (ICHD-II) defines criteria for CH as follows:

A. At least five attacks fulfilling criteria B to E
B. Severe or very severe unilateral, orbital, supraorbital, and/or temporal pain lasting 15 to 180 minutes if untreated
C. Headache is accompanied by at least one of the following:
   - Ipsilateral conjunctival injection and/or lacrimation
   - Ipsilateral nasal congestion and/or rhinorrhea
   - Ipsilateral eyelid edema
   - Ipsilateral forehead and facial sweating
   - Ipsilateral miosis and/or ptosis
   - A sense of restlessness or agitation
D. Attacks occur from one every other day to eight per day
E. Not attributed to another disorder

HISTORY AND EPIDEMIOLOGY

Although many clinicians have described CH over the centuries, Harris provided the first record of CH in the English literature in 1926, and Horton and colleagues provided the first comprehensive description of CH in 1939. Before CH became the accepted term, a large number of names were used to describe this unforgettable disorder (Table 14.1). Unlike migraine, CH is more common in men than women. Recent case series report male:female ratios between

TABLE 14.1 Historical Terms for CH

Ciliary neuralgia	Sluder's neuralgia
Horton's headache	Red migraine
Histaminic cephalalgia	Erythroprosopalgia of Bing
Petrosal neuralgia	Sphenopalatine neuralgia
Hemicrania periodic neuralgiforms	Autonomic faciocephalgia

Abbreviation: CH, cluster headache.

2.5 to 3.5:1. CH can begin at any age, but it most commonly begins in the second to fourth decade of life. The majority of CH sufferers are smokers, and may consume excessive coffee. About 4% of CH patients have a family history of CH, and CH is 5 to 18 times more common in first-degree relatives, suggesting a genetic influence for the disease.

CLINICAL FEATURES

CH exists in two forms. Episodic CH (ECH) patients experience periods of headache lasting from 1 week to 1 year, separated by periods without CH lasting for 1 month or more. Chronic CH (CCH) patients have attacks lasting for more than 1 year without remission or remissions lasting less than 1 month. Eighty to ninety percent of CH patients have ECH. About 10% of ECH patients transform to CCH, and about one third of CCH patients revert to ECH. The time length between cycles may increase as a patient ages.

CH is one of the most painful conditions encountered in clinical practice. The pain typically becomes maximally intense within 10 minutes. Attacks often occur with circadian patterns, often nocturnally about 1 to 2 hours after sleep. This suggests a correlation with the rapid eye movement (REM) sleep stage, and may be related to oxygen desaturation and obstructive sleep apnea in some patients. Common descriptions of pain include burning boring, or screwing, and sometimes throbbing or pulsating. Some patients report a feeling of a "hot poker in the eye." Some patients experience throbbing or pulsating pain. Some patients experience fluctuations of pain during an attack, and a few experience milder head pain between attacks. CH pain is typically located over the retro-orbital, supraorbital, or temporal area, but may occur in the jaw, cheek, teeth, ear, nose, or neck (Figure 14.1).

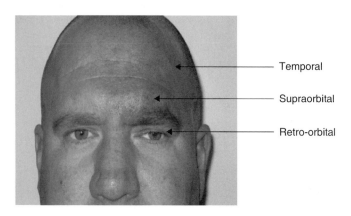

Temporal

Supraorbital

Retro-orbital

FIGURE 14.1 CH location.

CH patients typically experience attack cycles about twice a year to every 2 years, although some go many years between cycles. A typical cycle lasts 1 to 3 months, often with a seasonal pattern, with the cycle always beginning around the same month of the year. CH attacks tend to be milder at the beginning and near the end of a cycle.

Cranial autonomic symptoms, usually ipsilateral to the site of pain, are an obligatory feature of CH. The most common symptoms are lacrimation, conjunctival injection, and nasal congestion or rhinorrhea. Most symptoms are present only during attacks, but some patients, especially those with frequent attacks, experience a persistent partial Horner's syndrome (ptosis and/or miosis). Most CH patients feel a sense of restlessness or agitation during attacks, and pace or rock back and forth rather than lie down. Rarely do patients exhibit violent behavior, but the extreme nature of the pain has led some patients to take their own lives, hence the nickname "suicide headache."

TABLE 14.2 Migraine and CH Clinical Features

Clinical Features	Migraine	Cluster
Severe attacks	>4 hours	3 hours or less
Side	Unilateral or bilateral	Unilateral
Location	Frontal, occipital, orbital, temporal, cervical	Usually orbital
Character of pain	Usually throbbing/pulsating	Often boring, stabbing
Onset and cessation	Usually gradual	Rapid
Movement/activity	Worsens symptoms	May improve symptoms
Autonomic features	Occasionally	Always
More common in	Women	Men
Attacks triggered by alcohol	Common, but headache hours later	Almost always, often severe within minutes
Response to SC sumatriptan	Usually	Almost always
Response to high-flow oxygen	Uncommon	Usually
Seasonal attacks	Occasional	Common
Circadian periodicity	Uncommon	Very common
Comorbid conditions	Depression, anxiety, bipolar disease, epilepsy, Raynaud's syndrome, others	Tobacco abuse

Abbreviations: CH, cluster headache; SC, subcutaneous.

Migrainous symptoms are not rare in CH and may include premonitory symptoms, allodynia, nausea or vomiting, photophobia, phonophobia, or aura. Photophobia often occurs only ipsilateral to the site of pain. These symptoms may confuse the diagnosis of CH and migraine (Table 14.2).

As in migraine, CH attacks have a variety of triggers. Alcohol is the most common trigger, and many patients will experience severe attacks within minutes after drinking alcohol. Other common triggers are listed in Table 14.3.

TABLE 14.3 Common Triggers in CH

■ Alcohol	■ Nitroglycerin
■ Histamine	■ REM sleep
■ Exercise	■ Lack of sleep
■ Elevated temperature	

Abbreviation: CH, cluster headache.

PATHOPHYSIOLOGY

The pathophysiology of CH is not well understood, but it probably involves genetic, environmental, and chemical factors. The posterior hypothalamus, an important regulator of circadian cycles, appears important in CH, and positron emission tomography (PET) studies indicate activation during acute attacks (Figure 14.2).

As in migraine, activation of the trigeminovascular system and dilation of blood vessels occur during attacks, but the dilation is probably triggered

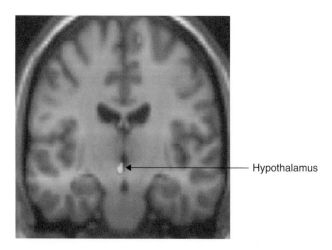

— Hypothalamus

FIGURE 14.2 Hypothalamic activation in CH as seen on PET.

in response to neuronal factors. Neuropeptides, including calcitonin gene-related peptide and vasoactive intestinal peptide, are elevated in acute attacks. Based on the presence of both sympathetic (forehead sweating, Horner's syndrome) and parasympathetic (lacrimation, congestion) symptoms, it seems likely that the autonomic system is activated in acute CH attacks.

A history of head trauma is common in CH, sometimes preceding CH by many years. Eye trauma, including enucleation of the ipsilateral eye, and dental extractions may precipitate CH. Hormonal factors, such as menstrual cycles, appear less important than they are in migraine, but it is worth noting that low testosterone is associated with CH in both genders.

DIFFERENTIAL DIAGNOSIS

Because several conditions can mimic CH, it may be reasonable to perform a magnetic resonance imaging study of all patients presenting with CH. Primary headaches that may resemble CH include migraine, hemicrania continua, hypnic headache, and the other TACs (Table 14.4). Secondary headaches that mimic CH include many ophthalmologic, vascular, infectious, and cervicomedullary disorders (Chapter 3). Many of these disorders have clinical features that distinguish them from CH.

ACUTE TREATMENT

CH attacks do not respond to many common headache treatments, such as over-the-counter or prescription medications (nonsteroidal anti-inflammatory drugs [NSAIDs], acetaminophen, opioids). Oral medications are usually not absorbed quickly enough to be effective.

The most effective medications for acute CH attacks are subcutaneous (SC) sumatriptan and 100% oxygen. SC sumatriptan 6 mg was effective within 15 minutes for over 90% of patients in clinical trials. Like other triptans, it should not be used by patients with ischemic heart disease or uncontrolled hypertension. Intranasal sumatriptan 20 mg and zolmitriptan 5 mg are also fairly effective, but with a slower onset of action and less efficacy.

Ergotamine and its derivative dihydroergotamine (DHE) are effective in acute CH. Because ergotamine can cause severe vasoconstriction, hypertension, and rarely liver or kidney disease, DHE is preferred. Intravenous (IV) DHE is most effective, but IM or NS may also work. Oxygen inhalation is effective in about 70% of CH attacks, with no known adverse events. The inhalation should be 100% oxygen at 10 to 15 liters/minute inhaled continuously for 15 minutes via a nonrebreathing face mask. Hyperbaric oxygen also appears effective, but has not proven more effective than normobaric oxygen.

TABLE 14.4 Selected CH Mimics

Condition	Distinguishing Features
Primary headaches	
Hemicrania continua	Continuous pain, autonomic symptoms, and less distinct attacks. Responsive to indomethacin but not triptans
Hypnic headache	Nocturnal but usually dull pain with no/mild autonomic symptoms
Paroxysmal hemicrania	Attacks short-lasting (30 minutes or less) and frequent. Responsive to indomethacin but not triptans
SUNCT	Attacks short-lasting (4 minutes or less) with up to hundreds of attacks/day
Ophthalmologic disorders	
Acute angle closure glaucoma	Severe conjunctival injection, poorly reactive pupil, mid-dilated, cloudy cornea, elevated intraocular pressure
Corneal erosion	Sharp pain, moderately injected, dull cornea, vision loss
Optic neuritis	Vision loss, afferent papillary defect
Vascular disorders	
Carotid/vertebral dissection	Thunderclap onset, facial pain, prominent Horner's syndrome (carotid), neck pain, cerebellar symptoms (vertebral)
Giant cell arteritis	Jaw claudication, polymyalgia rheumatica, amaurosis fugax, increased sedimentation rate and/or C-reactive protein
CNS vasculitis	Neurologic deficits; progressive, abnormal angiography
Pituitary tumors	Visual field loss, endocrine abnormalities (elevated prolactin)
Herpes zoster (V1)	Rash, severe allodynia, cranial nerve palsies
Chiari malformation	Valsalva or cough headache. Downbeat nystagmus

Abbreviations: CH, cluster headache; CNS, central nervous system; SUNCT, short-lasting unilateral neuralgiform headache with conjunctival injection and tearing.

Other treatments for acute CH include cocaine or lidocaine applications using a cotton swab in the area of the pterygopalatine fossa, intranasal lidocaine solution or spray, SC or infusions of somatostatin or octreotide, olanzapine, ergotamine, and DHE (Table 14.5).

TABLE 14.5 Acute CH Treatments

Treatment	Comments
Highly effective	
SC sumatriptan	Most effective in the majority of CH sufferers
Oxygen 100% 10 to 15 L/min	Works best early in attacks
Moderately effective	
Intranasal sumatriptan	Usually does not completely abort attacks
Intranasal zolmitriptan	Effective in about 30 minutes
SC octreotide 100 mg	Alternative to triptans, oxygen
Unproven effectiveness	
Intranasal lidocaine	Usually only modestly effective
Intranasal capsaicin	
Ergotamine	Slower onset of action, do not use with triptans. May be effective in short-term prophylaxis
DHE	IV formulation most effective
Olanzapine	2.5 to 10 mg. Highly sedating

Abbreviations: CH, cluster headache; DHE, dihyroergotamine; SC, subcutaneous.

TRANSITIONAL TREATMENT

CH cycles are short-lasting and severe, and transitional treatment offers relief in the weeks before prophylactic medications start to work. Sometimes these treatments can abort a cycle by themselves.

Corticosteroids are the most established transitional treatments for CH. Prednisone 10 to 80 mg/day and dexamethasone 4 to 8 mg/day for up to 21 days appear effective. However, adverse events, such as weight gain, hyperglycemia, hypertension, depression, and insomnia are common. Serious adverse events, including osteonecrosis of the femoral head and adrenal suppression, are more common with prolonged therapy (over 30 days), so the dose is usually tapered. Usually corticosteroids are used on a short-term basis in conjunction with other preventive medications that may take longer to become effective. CH often recurs after corticosteroids are tapered and discontinued (Table 14.6).

TABLE 14.6 Corticosteroids in CH

Drug	Sample Tapering Schedules
Prednisone	100 mg × 2 days, 80 mg × 2 days, 60 mg × 2 days, 40 mg × 2 days, 20 mg × 4 days; 80 mg × 3 days, 60 mg × 3 days, 40 mg × 3 days, 20 mg × 3 days
Dexamethasone	4 mg twice daily × 2 weeks, then 4 mg daily × 1 week

Abbreviation: CH, cluster headache.

DHE IV for up to 3 days is another short-term transitional treatment in CH, especially for intractable cases or those with significant triptan overuse. In some cases it can help CCH patients revert to ECH. With appropriate monitoring, patients may receive IV DHE for up to 7 days.

Greater occipital nerve blocks ipsilateral to the site of pain appear effective in some patients with ECH and CCH as an alternative short-term prophylactic treatment. Usually these injections are done with a combination of local anesthetics and corticosteroids, and the effect appears to last for 3 to 4 weeks in responders. A sphenopalatine ganglion block under endoscopy is an alternative treatment for drug-resistant CH.

The use of long-acting oral triptans (naratriptan, frovatriptan) on a regular basis may be useful for some patients as a transitional treatment

PROPHYLACTIC TREATMENT

Many of the prophylactic treatments used in migraine have efficacy in CH, but others, such as β-blockers, tricyclic antidepressants, and biofeedback, are not proven effective. Often the dose of prophylactic medication used for CH must be more than that used for migraine.

Verapamil is the preventive treatment of choice for most patients unless it is contraindicated or cycles are very short-lasting. The usual dose is 360 mg daily, but some patients may use close to 1 g/day. Short-acting and extended-release forms both appear effective, but the extended-release forms have lower bioavailability. Adverse events include constipation, edema, and fatigue, but the most important is arrhythmia due to slowing of atrioventricular node conduction. Bradycardia is common, as are first and second-degree heart block, and bundle branch block may occur. Monitor ECGs frequently, including when starting verapamil, before increasing doses, and 10 days after increasing doses.

Lithium is also effective in CH, often at concentrations lower than what is needed to treat bipolar disorder. The usual dose ranges from 600 to 1200 mg/day, and lithium 900 mg/day appears as effective as verapamil 360 mg/day. Adverse events, such as weakness, nausea, ataxia, confusion, tremor, and seizures are common, especially with increased plasma levels. Monitor thyroid and renal function prior to and during treatment and avoid the use of diuretics and NSAIDs.

Serotonergic agonists and antagonists are used occasionally for CH. Methysergide, an antagonist at serotonin 2A/C receptors and agonist of 1B/D receptors, appears effective in some patients, especially those with ECH. Adverse events include muscle cramps, abdominal pain, and nausea. Serious adverse events with prolonged use include vasoconstriction and fibrotic reaction (cardiac, retroperitoneal, and pulmonary) and require careful monitoring. These agents should be used for ECH patients with relatively short-lasting cycles. Methysergide is no longer available in the United States, but

TABLE 14.7 Selected Preventative Medications in CH

Medication	Daily Dose (mg)	Comments
Verapamil	120–960	Monitoring ECG is essential
Lithium	600–1200	Adjust for serum level of 1 mmol/L
Topiramate	25–200	Usually effective in 4 weeks or less in CH
Gabapentin	900–1800	May be useful in refractory CH, allodynia
Valproic acid	500–2000	May need to use higher doses in CH (levels up to 120). Useful in CCH
Melatonin	9–24	Use at night
Ergotamine	2–3	Given at night for nocturnal CH
DHE	1–3	IV for refractory CH (after an antiemetic)
Methysergide	3–12	Avoid prolonged use
Leuprolide	3.75 (once)	Decreased libido most common adverse event

Abbreviations: CH, cluster headache; DHE, dihyroergotamine.

methylergonovine, a derivative of methysergide, may be effective for some CH patients. Leuprolide, a synthetic, slow-release, gonadotropin-releasing hormone analogue, appeared to be effective in reducing intensity and length of CH attacks in one placebo-controlled trial.

Anticonvulsants, including valproic acid, topiramate, and gabapentin, appear to have some effect in open-label studies but have not been established in larger placebo-controlled studies. These agents are attractive alternatives for patients with a poor/inadequate response or contraindications to verapamil. Some patients may find melatonin, important in circadian rhythms, to be effective at high doses (9 mg or more) as an adjunctive agent. Intranasal capsaicin, or civamide, a capsaicin analog, appear effective in a subset of CH patients, including those with CCH. Sodium oxybate may be effective for patients with strictly nocturnal, refractory attacks (Table 14.7).

REFRACTORY CH

With effective preventive and acute medication, CH usually has a favorable treatment outcome. But in some cases, CH may be refractory to the usual treatment measures and it is worth considering other treatment options or reasons for treatment failure (Table 14.8).

Although medication overuse is most common in migraine, there appears to be a subset of CH patients (who may have coexistent migraine) who experience medication overuse headache (MOH) with increasing medication use. Triptans are the medications most commonly overused by CH patients, but the

TABLE 14.8 Strategies for Refractory CH

- Increase dose of prophylactic medication
- Address other medical problems (i.e., sleep apnea)
- Use more than one preventive
- Address medication overuse if present (triptans, opioids)
- Repetitive DHE
- Greater occipital nerve blockade
- Neuromodulatory procedures

Abbreviations: CH, cluster headache; DHE, dihyroergotamine.

headaches may respond to withdrawal and short-term prophylaxis with corticosteroids or IV DHE. Opioids and combination analgesics may also cause MOH in patients with CH, and long-term opioid use for CH should generally be avoided. CH patients appear particularly susceptible to MOH if they have a personal or family history of migraine.

Neuromodulatory procedures have great promise but also carry significant risks. In open-label studies, occipital nerve stimulation reduced the intensity and frequency of CH attacks in most subjects. Some subjects experienced relatively rapid recurrence when their devices malfunctioned or the stimulation was turned off. There is now a consensus that this is the preferred treatment for

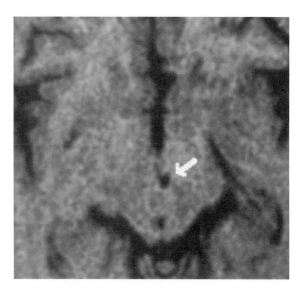

FIGURE 14.3 Deep brain stimulation in CH (arrow shows an electrode in the left posterior hypothalamus).

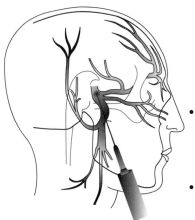

• Sensory trigeminal pathway
  procedures
  • Radiofrequency or glycerol rhizotomy
  • Gamma knife radiosurgery
  • Trigeminal root section
  • Other
• Autonomic (parasympathetic)
  pathway procedures

FIGURE 14.4 Destructive surgeries for refractory CH.

refractory CH. Patients can receive greater occipital and supraorbital stimulation together, which in our experience gives the best result. Deep brain stimulation of the posterior hypothalamus can provide substantial improvement (Figure 14.3), but one patient in the initial study died of implantation-induced intracranial hemorrhage. Destructive surgeries, such as trigeminal sensory rhizotomy, microvascular decompression of the trigeminal nerve, or gamma knife radiotherapy, may result in diplopia, corneal anesthesia, or anesthesia dolorosa and should only be undertaken as a last resort (Figure 14.4).

REFERENCES

Donnet A, Lanteri-Minet M, Guegan-Massardier E, et al. Chronic cluster headache: a French clinical descriptive study. *J Neurol Neurosurg Psychiatry*. 2007;78:1354–1358.

May A, Bahra A, Buchel C, Frackowiak RS, Goadsby PJ. Hypothalamic activation in cluster headache attacks. *Lancet*. 1998;352:275–278.

Peatfield R. Migrainous features in cluster headache. *Curr Pain Headache Rep*. 2001;5(1):67–70.

Rozen T. Trigeminal autonomic cephalalgias. *Continuum Headache*. 2006;6:171–193.

Schürks M, Rosskopf D, de Jesus J, et al. Predictors of acute treatment response among patients with cluster headache. *Headache*. 2007;47(7):1079–1084.

15 Unusual Primary Headaches

Most patients who present to a headache center have a primary headache disorder that is not attributable to another disorder. Migraine headache, tension-type headache, and trigeminal autonomic cephalgias (TAC, i.e., cluster headache [CH], paroxysmal hemicrania [PH], short-lasting unilateral neuralgiform headache with conjunctival injection and tearing [SUNCT], and short-lasting unilateral neuralgiform headache with cranial autonomic features [SUNA]) make up the majority of primary headaches seen in clinical practice. Experienced clinicians should become adept at recognizing these and other uncommon primary headache disorders (Table 15.1). After excluding secondary headache disorders, use clinical features to distinguish between the various primary headaches (Table 15.2).

LONG-LASTING PRIMARY HEADACHE DISORDERS

Chronic daily headache (CDH) is defined as headache lasting 4 or more hours on 15 or more days a month. In population-based studies, about 4% to 5% of people have CDH, and CDH is the most common presentation in tertiary headache clinics. Excluding secondary headache disorders, chronic migraine and chronic tension-type headache are the most common causes of CDH. However, new daily persistent headache and hemicrania continua (HC) are not rare and may be misdiagnosed (Chapter 8).

TABLE 15.1 Notable Primary Headache Disorders

■ Migraine (episodic or chronic)	■ Tension-type headache
■ TACs	■ New daily persistent headache
• Cluster (episodic or chronic)	■ Hypnic headache
• Paroxysmal hemicrania	■ Hemicrania continua
• SUNCT/SUNA	■ Primary thunderclap headache
■ Primary cough headache	■ Primary stabbing headache
■ Headache associated with sexual activity	■ Primary exertional headache
■ Nummular headache	■ Trigeminal neuralgia
■ Burning mouth syndrome	■ Atypical facial pain

Abbreviations: SUNA, short-lasting unilateral neuralgiform headache with cranial autonomic features; SUNCT, short-lasting unilateral neuralgiform headache with conjunctival injection and tearing; TACs, trigeminal autonomic cephalalgia.

TABLE 15.2 Primary Headache Disorders

Chronic daily headache
   Chronic migraine
   Chronic tension-type headache
   Hemicrania continua
   New daily persistent headache
Short-duration, triggered headache
   Cough headache, exertional headache, sexual headache
Short-duration, nontriggered headache
   Tension headache, cluster headache, hypnic headache,
      paroxysmal hemicrania, SUNCT
Headache lasting 4+ hours
   Migraine headache, tension-type headache
Facial Pain
   Trigeminal neuralgia, atypical facial pain, burning mouth syndrome

Abbreviations: SUNCT, short-lasting unilateral neuralgiform headache with conjunctival injection and tearing.

SHORT-LASTING, TRIGGERED PRIMARY HEADACHE DISORDERS

Primary Cough Headache

Primary cough headache (Table 15.3) is a sudden-onset headache triggered by coughing, sneezing, straining, or Valsalva maneuvers. The pain is usually bilateral, often stabbing or sharp, and located at the vertex, frontal, or temporal area. Most patients deny neurologic symptoms, and migraine features are uncommon.

The cause of the pain of primary cough headache may be the effect of sudden increases of intracranial pressure causing irritation of the cerebellar tonsils. Primary cough headache is most common in patients more than age 40. About one-half of cough headaches are because of secondary causes, such as vascular disease, Chiari malformations, cerebral aneurysms, or brain tumors, especially in the posterior fossa (Figure 15.1). Indomethacin and lumbar puncture may alleviate both primary and secondary cough headaches.

TABLE 15.3 ICHD-II Criteria for Primary Cough Headache

- Sudden onset lasting 1 second to 30 minutes
- Brought on by and occurring only in association with coughing, straining, and/or Valsalva maneuver
- Not attributed to another disorder

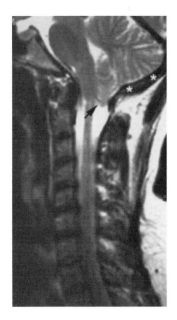

FIGURE 15.1 Cough headache associated with Chiari malformation. *Source*: From Pascual J. Activity-related headache. In: Gilman S, ed. *MedLink Neurology*. San Diego, CA: MedLink Corporation.

Primary Exertional Headache

Exertional headaches (Table 15.4) are not rare, and they are especially common in younger patients. The pain is often throbbing or pulsatile, usually bilateral, and lasts 5 minutes to 48 hours. High temperature and humidity can worsen symptoms. Many patients have a personal or family history of migraine. Patients may pretreat with pain medication, such as indomethacin, before exertion, or slowly increase their activity level before more significant exertion. In most cases, primary exertional headache is self-limiting with improvement occurring after 3 to 6 months. As with cough headache, clinicians should exclude secondary causes.

TABLE 15.4 ICHD-II Criteria for Primary Exertional Headache

Diagnostic criteria
- Lasting from 5 minutes to 48 hours
- Brought on by and occurring only during or after physical exertion
- Not attributed to another disorder

Primary Headache Associated with Sexual Activity

Headache associated with sexual activity (Table 15.5) is more common in men than women and can be preorgasmic or orgasmic. Orgasmic headaches are more common, and clinicians must exclude secondary headaches, such as subarachnoid hemorrhage or arterial dissection, at first onset. Orgasmic headaches are often severe and last anywhere from 1 minute to 3 hours. After excluding secondary causes, the headaches may be relieved with pre-emptive treatment, such as triptans or indomethacin. Preorgasmic headaches are less common and usually start as a dull bilateral ache that worsens as sexual excitement increases. Some feel that orgasmic headache is a variant of migraine and preorgasmic headache is related to chronic tension-type headache. Headaches related to sexual activity are unpredictable and may resolve without treatment. Pre-emptive treatment with indomethacin or triptans and preventative medication may be useful in some patients.

TABLE 15.5 ICHD-II Criteria for Primary Headache Associated with Sexual Activity

Preorgasmic Headache	Orgasmic Headache
Diagnostic criteria:	Diagnostic criteria:
A. Dull ache in the head and neck associated with awareness of neck and/or jaw muscle contraction and fulfilling criterion B	A. Sudden, severe ("explosive") headache fulfilling criterion B
B. Occurs during sexual activity and increases with sexual excitement	B. Occurs at orgasm
C. Not attributed to another disorder	C. Not attributed to another disorder

SHORT-LASTING, NONTRIGGERED PRIMARY HEADACHE DISORDERS

TACs (Table 15.6) are relatively common causes of short-lasting (< 4 hours) primary headaches. CH (Chapter 14) is the most common type of TAC, whereas PH, SUNCT, and SUNA are relatively rare. As with CH, autonomic symptoms are prominent and the hypothalamus appears to be involved, but TAC attacks are shorter and more frequent. TACs (including CH) have multiple potential secondary causes (Chapter 3), and it is difficult to determine if headaches are primary or secondary based on clinical criteria. Obtaining magnetic resonance imaging (MRI) with dedicated pituitary sequences in all patients with TACs may be necessary.

TABLE 15.6 Clinical Characteristics of the TACs

Disorder	Duration	Frequency	Location	Character	Migraine Features?	Gender (F:M)
CH	15–180 minutes	Every other day to 8 per day	Orbital, frontal, temporal	Very severe, boring	Sometimes	1:3–7
PH	2–30 minutes	1–40 per day	Orbital, frontal, temporal	Very severe, boring, throbbing	Sometimes	2–3:1
SUNA	2–600 seconds	Dozens to hundreds per day	Orbital, frontal	Very severe, burning, stabbing	Sometimes	2:1
SUNCT	5–240 seconds	Dozens to hundreds per day	Orbital, frontal	Very severe, burning, stabbing	No	1:2

Abbreviations: CH, cluster headache; PH, paroxysmal hemicrania; SUNA, short-lasting unilateral neuralgiform headache with cranial autonomic features; SUNCT, short-lasting unilateral neuralgiform headache with conjunctival injection and tearing.

TABLE 15.7 ICHD-II Criteria for Paroxysmal Hemicrania

Diagnostic criteria:
A. At least 20 attacks fulfilling criteria B–D
B. Attacks of severe, unilateral, orbital, supraorbital, or temporal pain lasting 2–30 minutes
C. Headache is accompanied by at least one of the following:
    1. Ipsilateral conjunctival injection and/or lacrimation
    2. Ipsilateral nasal congestion and/or rhinorrhea
    3. Ipsilateral eyelid edema
    4. Ipsilateral forehead and facial sweating
    5. Ipsilateral miosis and/or ptosis
D. Attacks have a frequency above 5 per day for more than half of the time, although periods with lower frequency may occur
E. Attacks are prevented completely by therapeutic doses of indomethacin
F. Not attributed to another disorder

Paroxysmal Hemicrania

PH (Table 15.7) is a rare TAC characterized by attacks that are more frequent but shorter-lasting, less severe, and less likely to cause agitation than CH. PH is more common in women than men. PH is an indomethacin-responsive headache disorder and does not respond to triptans or oxygen. Some patients with PH experience pain between attacks, but the attacks are more discrete than those of HC. Unlike CH, most patients have a chronic form without remissions, but some patients experience remissions of 1 month or more. If indomethacin is not tolerated, selective cyclooxygenase-2 inhibitors such as celecoxib or calcium channel blockers may be effective. As with CH, secondary headaches may mimic PH and neuroimaging is recommended for all patients with TACs. Some causes of symptomatic PH include the following:

■ Vascular disorders (circle of Willis aneurysm, middle cerebral artery infarct, arteriovenous malformation)
■ Tumors (frontal lobe, pituitary, cavernous sinus meningioma)
■ Ophthalmic herpes zoster
■ Trauma
■ Dental pathology

Indomethacin-Responsive Headaches

PH is an indomethacin-responsive headache disorder that is diagnosed only when patients respond absolutely to indomethacin. Like other nonsteroidal

TABLE 15.8 Possible Indomethacin-Responsive Headache Disorders

Hemicrania continua[a]	Paroxysmal hemicrania[a]
Primary cough headache	Primary headache associated with sexual activity
Cluster headache	Idiopathic stabbing headache ("ice-pick" or "jabs and jolts")

[a] A complete response to indomethacin is required for the diagnosis.

TABLE 15.9 Tips for Prescribing an Indomethacin Trial

- Start at 25 mg three times daily or extended release 75 mg once a day for 3 to 7 days
- If tolerated but no response, increase up to 225 mg/day
- Use antacids, histamine receptor antagonists, or proton pump inhibitors to reduce adverse events in patients receiving long-term therapy
- Use the extended release form in the evening to prevent nocturnal symptoms
- Some patients require a higher dose (up to 300 mg/day) for best effect
- Avoid skipping doses, especially in the titration phase
- If patients respond, occasionally attempt to lower the dose after stabilization
- Counsel patients that indomethacin should be effective in less than 1 month—if it is not helpful by then it should be discontinued
- Address acute medication overuse, if present. Opioids may decrease the response to NSAID therapy

Abbreviation: NSAID, nonsteroidal anti-inflammatory drug.

anti-inflammatory drugs (NSAIDs), indomethacin inhibits cyclooxygenase (predominantly cox-1), thus inhibiting synthesis of prostaglandins, a mediator of inflammation. It is not clear why indomethacin is more effective than other NSAIDs for many headache disorders, but it could be because of its structural similarities to serotonin, central vasoconstrictive and analgesic properties, or lowering of intracranial pressure. It also inhibits the metabolism of an active progesterone metabolite.

A number of primary headache disorders may respond to treatment with indomethacin as listed in Table 15.8.

When an indomethacin-responsive headache disorder is suspected, start indomethacin at low doses and increase every few days until improvement or side effects occur. Tips for the use of indomethacin in a daily trial are listed in Table 15.9.

SUNCT and SUNA

SUNCT and SUNA are typified by severe, brief, unilateral attacks that usually occur in the distribution of the trigeminal nerve. Patients describe the pain as stabbing, burning, prickling, piercing, shooting, or like an electric shock.

TABLE 15.10 ICHD-II Criteria for SUNCT and SUNA

SUNCT	SUNA
A. At least 20 attacks fulfilling criteria B–D	A. At least 20 attacks fulfilling criteria B–E
B. Attacks of unilateral, orbital, supraorbital, or temporal stabbing or pulsating pain lasting 5–240 seconds	B. Attacks of unilateral, orbital, supraorbital, or temporal stabbing or pulsating pain lasting from 2 seconds to 10 minutes
C. Pain is accompanied by ipsilateral conjunctival injection and lacrimation	C. Pain is accompanied by one of: 1. Conjunctival injection and/or lacrimation 2. Nasal congestion and/or rhinorrhea 3. Eyelid edema
D. Attack frequency is 3 to 200 per day	D. Attack frequency is ≥1 per day for more than half of the time
E. Not attributed to another disorder	E. No refractory period follows attacks triggered from trigger areas
	F. Not attributed to another disorder

Abbreviations: SUNA, short-lasting unilateral neuralgiform headache with cranial autonomic features; SUNCT, short-lasting unilateral neuralgiform headache with conjunctival injection and tearing.

SUNA differs from SUNCT in that autonomic symptoms are less prominent (Table 15.10).

SUNCT or SUNA may be confused with trigeminal neuralgia (TN) in patients with brief headache or facial pain (Figure 15.2). Most patients with

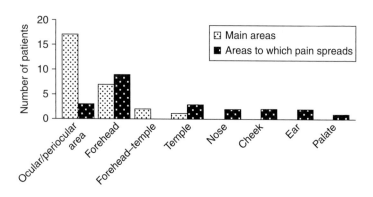

FIGURE 15.2 Pain location in SUNCT.

TABLE 15.11 Prophylactic Treatments for SUNCT and SUNA

Medication	Daily Dose
IV lidocaine	1–4 mg/min infusion
Lamotrigine	100–400 mg
Gabapentin	800–2700 mg
Topiramate	50–300 mg
Carbamazepine	400–1200 mg

Abbreviations: IV, intravenous; SUNA, short-lasting unilateral neuralgiform headache with cranial autonomic features; SUNCT, short-lasting unilateral neuralgiform headache with conjunctival injection and tearing.

SUNCT describe pain that begins in the ocular or forehead area, whereas TN pain is more common in the V2 area. Unlike TN, most SUNCT attacks are often spontaneous and not triggered by other stimuli. SUNCT and SUNA patients do not usually experience a refractory period: one attack may occur immediately following another. Numbness or allodynia in the affected area is not rare. As with other TACs, multiple causes of secondary SUNCT have been reported, including pituitary tumors and posterior fossa abnormalities, but unlike TN, evidence of a vascular loop on MRI is uncommon (about 7%).

Because of the short-lasting nature of SUNCT and SUNA attacks, prophylaxis is the mainstay of treatment for these disorders. Patients can experience up to 30 attacks/hour. The most effective treatment for short-term prevention is intravenous lidocaine. In case series, most patients had at least a partial response, usually in a few days or less, with many experiencing pain-free periods of weeks or months. Lamotrigine is the first-line agent for long-term prevention, but many other treatments have shown promise based on open-label studies. As with CH, invasive surgical procedures and hypothalamic stimulation should be reserved for refractory patients (Table 15.11).

Hypnic Headache

Hypnic or "alarm-clock" headache (Table 15.12) is a sleep-related primary headache disorder most common in elderly patients. The pain usually begins between 1:00 and 3:00 am, with an abrupt onset of bilateral, throbbing, anterior pain. The pain is sometimes unilateral, occipital, or associated with autonomic features, and usually resolves in 1 to 2 hours.

Polysomnography suggests that hypnic headache develops during rapid eye movement sleep, and serotonin and melatonin dysregulation may be important in its pathophysiology. Rule out a secondary cause, such as nocturnal

TABLE 15.12 ICHD-II Criteria for Hypnic Headache

A. Dull headache fulfilling criteria B–D
B. Develops only during sleep, and awakens patient
C. At least two of the following characteristics:
    1. Occurs >15 times per month
    2. Lasts ≥15 minutes after waking
    3. First occurs after age 50
D. No autonomic symptoms and no more than one of nausea, photophobia, or phonophobia
E. Not attributed to another disorder

hypertension or obstructive sleep apnea, with new-onset hypnic headache. A sleep study and neuroimaging may be necessary.

Lithium (300–600 mg) is an effective prophylactic treatment, but it is poorly tolerated. Some patients find caffeine (40–60 mg) and high-dose melatonin useful. Case reports suggest that flunarizine 5 mg, indomethacin 25 to 75 mg, and topiramate 25 to 100 mg at night are effective.

Nummular Headache

Nummular headache was previously called "coin-shaped cephalgia." Patients usually describe a focal, circumscribed area of mild, moderate, or severe pain with variable pain characteristics. Some postulate that nummular headache is a symptom of irritation of a terminal branch of a sensory nerve. The majority of patients have chronic pain, and sensory symptoms (paresthesias, hyperesthesias) are more common than migrainous symptoms. At least half of patients benefit from injection of onabotulinumtoxinA in a grid pattern over the area of pain. One advantage of onabotulinumtoxinA is that patients often respond to relatively low doses (often less than 25 units) and can avoid undesirable side effects from preventative medication.

TABLE 15.13 ICHD-II Criteria for Primary Stabbing Headache

A. Head pain occurring as a single stab or a series of stabs and fulfilling criteria B–D
B. Exclusively or predominantly felt in the distribution of the first division of the trigeminal nerve (orbit, temple, and parietal areas)
C. Stabs last for up to a few seconds and recur with irregular frequency ranging from one to many per day
D. No accompanying symptoms
E. Not attributed to another disorder

Primary (Idiopathic) Stabbing Headache

Primary stabbing headache (Table 15.13) usually coexists with other primary headache disorders. Most attacks are brief, unilateral, and last 1 to 10 seconds. Attacks commonly occur in the orbital, temporal, parietal, and occipital areas. Most patients do not experience clear triggers or autonomic features. Many patients respond to indomethacin 25 to 150 mg/day.

Primary Thunderclap Headache

Thunderclap or sudden-onset headache (Table 15.14) requires an extensive work-up, including neuroimaging, lumbar puncture, and, at times, angiography, for secondary causes (Chapter 3). Often no cause is found, and patients can be diagnosed with primary thunderclap headache. Primary thunderclap headache may precede or follow a diagnosis of migraine. Exertion and hyperventilation may provoke attacks. The occipital region is the most common site of pain, which often lingers for days after onset. Primary thunderclap headache may be related to reversible cerebral vasoconstriction syndrome (e.g., Call-Fleming syndrome), but patients with primary thunderclap headache do not have segmental vasoconstriction on angiography.

TABLE 15.14 ICHD-II Criteria for Primary Thunderclap Headache

A. Severe head pain fulfilling criteria B and C
B. Both of the following characteristics:
    1. Sudden onset, reaching maximum intensity in <1 minute
    2. Lasting from 1 hour to 10 days
C. Does not recur regularly over subsequent weeks or months
D. Not attributed to another disorder

Ophthalmoplegic Migraine

Ophthalmoplegic migraine (Table 15.15) refers to recurrent attacks of headache with migrainous characteristics associated with paresis of one or more

TABLE 15.15 ICHD-II Criteria for Ophthalmoplegic "Migraine"

A. At least two attacks fulfilling criterion B
B. Migraine-like headache accompanied or followed within 4 days of its onset by paresis of one or more of the third, fourth, and/or sixth cranial nerves
C. Parasellar, orbital fissure, and posterior fossa lesions ruled out by appropriate investigations

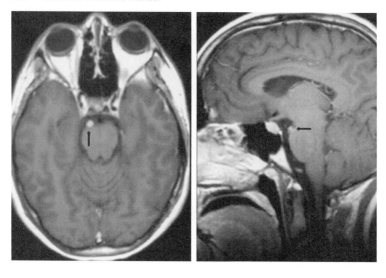

FIGURE 15.3 Right oculomotor nerve enhancement in a pediatric patient with ophthalmoplegic migraine.
Source: Brarucha et al., *Pediatric Neurology*. 2007.

ocular cranial nerves. The third (oculomotor) nerve is the most commonly affected. Previously thought to be a variant of migraine, it is now characterized as a recurrent demyelinating neuropathy based on MRI findings that show gadolinium enhancement of the affected nerve (Figure 15.3). Headaches are long-lasting (often more than a week) and some patients have a latent period of 4 days between headache onset and ophthalmoplegia. The condition is more common in children than adults.

Facial Pain

Cranial neuralgias and facial pain may be primary or secondary and often are disabling. Although TN is the most well-understood disorder associated with facial pain, we will review some other important causes of facial pain.

Trigeminal neuralgia

TN (Table 15.16) is a painful disorder of the face characterized by short-lasting electric pain in one or more divisions of the trigeminal nerve. Characteristics that distinguish TN from other causes of facial pain, such as SUNCT or primary stabbing headache, include the following:

- Attacks often triggered by touch, chewing, talking, brushing teeth, or emotional distress
- Pain usually starts in a small trigger zone

TABLE 15.16 ICHD-II Criteria for Classic Trigeminal Neuralgia

A. Paroxysmal attacks of pain lasting from a fraction of a second to 2 minutes, affecting one or more divisions of the trigeminal nerve and fulfilling criteria B and C
B. Pain has at least one of the following characteristics:
  1. Intense, sharp, superficial, or stabbing
  2. Precipitated from trigger areas or by trigger factors
C. Attacks are stereotyped in the individual patient
D. No clinically evident neurologic deficit
E. Not attributed to another disorder (other than microvascular compression)

- Most patients experience a refractory period after stimulation, especially after severe attacks
- Most attacks occur in the V2 or V3 distribution
- Patients may freeze and grimace with facial contortions (tic douloureux) with attacks

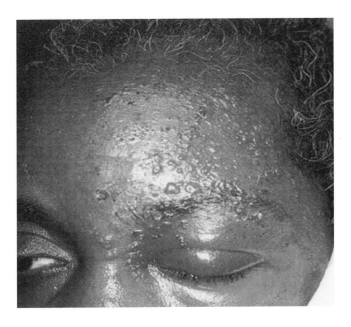

FIGURE 15.4 Herpes zoster.
Source: SKINmed, 2003 Le Jacq Communications.

The cause of "classic" TN is microvascular compression of the trigeminal nerve by a vascular loop (usually the superior cerebellar artery) producing a chronic focal demyelination of the trigeminal nerve. Progressive symptoms and facial numbness may be more likely to suggest a secondary cause, such as neoplasm, brainstem infarct, infection such as herpes zoster (Figure 15.4), or syringobulbia. Demyelinating disease, such as multiple sclerosis, may cause TN and should be suspected in young patients or those with bilateral disease. Vasoactive intestinal peptide appears elevated in acute TN attacks and may enhance the effect of substance P, leading to pain.

TABLE 15.17 Medications in the Treatment of TN

Medication	Daily Maintenance Dose
Carbamazepine	200–800 mg
Phenytoin	200–500 mg
Baclofen	30–60 mg
Clonazepam	1.5–8 mg
Gabapentin	900–2400 mg
Oxycarbamazepine	900–1800 mg
Topiramate	100–300 mg
Onabotulinumtoxin Type A	Up to 25 units/q3 months

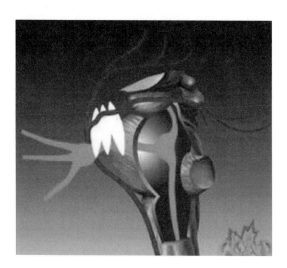

FIGURE 15.5 Microvascular decompression.
Source: http://www.umanitoba.ca/cranial_nerves/trigeminal_neuralgia/microvascular_decompression_surgery.html

Treatment of TN includes medication (Table 15.17) and surgery for refractory cases. Carbamazepine is the first-line and most studied medication, but many other medications have been used, with some success. Constant pain between attacks predicts a worse prognosis.

Medications for the treatment of TN may become less effective over time, and up to 50% of patients eventually require surgical treatment. Microvascular decompression to remove the vessel compressing the nerve is usually effective, with 80% of patients having complete postoperative pain relief and the majority remaining pain-free for a decade. Microvascular decompression has a larger number of significant risks, including hearing loss, stroke, or death, than do peripheral procedures (Figure 15.5).

Other surgical options include radiofrequency rhizotomy, balloon compression, gamma knife radiosurgery, peripheral denervation with alcohol, cutting or freezing the nerve, and onabotulinumtoxinA injection into the areas of pain. The benefits of these treatments do not last as long as microvascular decompression. The principles of TN management are as follows:

- Use low doses of medication whenever possible (many of the effective medications are not well tolerated by elderly patients)
- Remember that medication responsiveness changes over time
- Consider polytherapy
- Consider intravenous phenytoin or fosphenytoin for emergency room use
- Attempt to taper the medication after prolonged pain-free periods
- Be aware that many patients will eventually require surgical procedures
- Choose surgical procedures based in part on disability and life-expectancy.

Glossopharyngeal neuralgia

Glossopharyngeal neuralgia (Table 15.18) is characterized by pain in the throat, tonsils, ear, and tongue that lasts less than 1 minute and is triggered

TABLE 15.18 ICHD-II Criteria for Glossopharyngeal Neuralgia

A. Paroxysmal attacks of facial pain lasting from a fraction of a second to 2 minutes and fulfilling criteria B and C
B. Pain has all of the following characteristics:
    1. Unilateral location
    2. Distribution within the posterior part of the tongue, tonsillar fossa, pharynx, or beneath the angle of the lower jaw and/or in the ear
    3. Sharp, stabbing, and severe
    4. Precipitated by swallowing, chewing, talking, coughing, and/or yawning
C. Attacks are stereotyped in the individual patient
D. No clinically evident neurologic deficit
E. Not attributed to another disorder

TABLE 15.19 ICHD-II Criteria for Persistent Idiopathic Facial Pain

A. Pain in the face, present daily and persisting for all or most of the day, fulfilling criteria B and C
B. Pain is confined at onset to a limited area on one side of the face, and is deep and poorly localized
C. Pain is not associated with sensory loss or other physical signs
D. Investigations including x-ray of face and jaws do not demonstrate any relevant abnormality

by swallowing. Syncope may accompany acute attacks. Many of the medications used for TN are effective for glossopharyngeal neuralgia. If response to these medications is inadequate, sectioning of the glossopharyngeal nerve and upper rootlets of the vagus nerve or microvascular decompression of the glossopharyngeal nerve may be effective.

Burning mouth syndrome
Burning mouth syndrome, characterized by a burning sensation in one or several oral structures, is most common in postmenopausal women. Fungal infections, such as candida, can cause burning mouth, as can contact allergies, oral infections, or reflux. Clonazepam tablets (0.5–1 mg three times daily) can be used topically without swallowing (chew, swish for several minutes, then spit).

Persistent idiopathic facial pain
Persistent idiopathic facial pain (Table 15.19), previously referred to as atypical facial pain, refers to types of facial pain that do not fit a classifiable pain syndrome. Patients with idiopathic facial pain often try to obtain relief with acute and preventive therapies and undergo multiple dental, nasal, or sinus procedures with no improvement. Patients are usually younger than those with TN, and affective disorders such as depression are common. While defined as featureless and poorly localized pain, migrainous symptoms are not rare, and patients may respond to migraine medications. Occasionally migraine will present with predominant facial pain, which we call "lower half" migraine. Treatments for neuropathic pain are occasionally helpful, but surgical procedures are less effective than in TN. Dental conditions, microabscesses, neoplasms of the face, and even lung carcinomas are among the reported causes of persistent idiopathic facial pain.

CONCLUSION

The management of facial pain can be challenging. Many patients require coordination of care among multiple providers including, neurology, oral surgery, pain management, psychology, and neurosurgery.

REFERENCES

Chen SP, Fuh JL, Lirng JF, Chang FC, Wang SJ. Recurrent primary thunderclap headache and benign CNS angiopathy: spectra of the same disorder? *Neurology*. 2006;67(12):2164–2169.

Graff-Radford SB. Facial pain. *Neurologist*. 2009;15(4):171–177.

Pascual J. Other primary headaches. *Neurol Clin*. 2009;27(2):557–571.

Queiroz LP. Symptoms and therapies: exertional and sexual headaches. *Curr Pain Headache Rep*. 2001;3:275–278.

Rozen TD. Trigeminal autonomic cephalalgias. *Neurol Clin*. 2009;27(2):537–556.

16 Posttraumatic Headache

Concussion is a trauma-induced alteration in mental status that may or may not involve loss of consciousness. Minor traumatic brain injury is a mechanically induced physiological disruption of brain function with any loss of consciousness, any anterograde or retrograde amnesia, any alteration in mental state at the time of the accident, or transient or persistent focal neurologic deficits.

The International Headache Society divides posttraumatic headache (PTH) based on the significance of the head trauma. The four factors that define significant head trauma are: (1) loss of consciousness lasting more than 30 minutes; (2) Glasgow coma scale of <13; (3) posttraumatic amnesia for 48 hours or more; and (4) abnormal imaging (brain, or skull fracture). According to the definition; symptoms must begin within 7 days of the injury. Usually they evolve seamlessly out of the original injury or start within 3 to 4 days. However, patients may not recall the exact time of onset, especially if there were other injuries and the use of pain medications early on. Acute PTH is headache that lasts less than 3 months; chronic PTH lasts longer.

Postconcussion (or posttraumatic) syndrome requires cognitive deficit and has at least three of the following eight symptoms: fatigue, sleep disturbance, headache, dizziness, irritability, affective disturbance, personality change, and apathy (Table 16.1). The symptoms begin or worsen after the injury. There is interference with social functioning. Dementia should be excluded.

TABLE 16.1 Nonheadache Symptoms

Cranial Nerve Symptoms and Signs	Psychologic and Somatic Complaints	Seizure-like Spells (EEG Usually Normal)
■ Dizziness	■ Irritability	■ Nonspecific staring episodes
■ Vertigo	■ Anxiety	■ Nonvestibular dizziness
■ Tinnitus	■ Depression	■ Periodic loss of consciousness
■ Hearing loss	■ Personality change	■ Narcolepsy- or cataplexy-like spells
■ Blurred vision	■ Fatigue	■ Episodic disorientation
■ Diplopia	■ Sleep disturbance	■ Fugue-like states
■ Convergence insufficiency	■ Decreased libido	
■ Light and noise sensitivity	■ Decreased appetite	
■ Diminished taste and smell		

Abbreviation: EEG, electroencephalogram.

Postconcussion syndrome (PCS) has been controversial for generations. In 1908, Harvey Cushing stated, "Although no objective signs accompany these complaints, they are so uniform from case to case that the symptoms cannot be regarded as other than genuine." This controversy continues and is fueled by the medicolegal system, which demands simplistic explanations and compensates doctors for overlisting and undertreating patients. Currently, there is less tendency to support the concept that most patients are malingering or another nonbiological explanation because PCS is so common among head-injured soldiers.

PTH may resemble chronic tension-type headache, migraine, chronic migraine, and cluster headache. Some patients with PTH have characteristics of multiple headache disorders. For cluster headache, in our experience, the original headache is not cluster-like, and the characteristic headache evolves out of the more nondescript acute PTH. Nonheadache symptoms are present in PCS and are listed in Table 16.1.

PTHs are common. One month after the emergency department (ED) visit for concussion 31% to 90% of patients complain of headache; 2 to 3 months after the ED visit 32% to 78% of patients complain of headache; 1 year after the ED visit 8% to 35% complain; and 2 to 4 years later 20% to 24%. Patients often do not spontaneously admit to headache, dizziness, depression, anxiety, and irritability. Patients must be questioned directly about these symptoms.

Other traumatically induced headaches may occur, including headaches related to:

■ Subdural/epidural hematoma
■ Intracranial hypotension
■ Intracranial hypertension
■ Cervicogenic headache
■ Dysautonomic cephalgia
■ Styloid process fracture
■ Temporomandibular joint injury

Head trauma results in complex and chaotic brain motion. This causes immediate disruption of brain function with the extracellular release of calcium, potassium, and glutamate and more prolonged metabolic alteration in glucose metabolism and blood flow (Figure 16.1).

Diffusion tensor imaging may show reduced white matter integrity from diffuse axonal injury in the anterior corona radiata, uncinate fasciculus, corpus callosum, inferior longitudinal fasciculus, and cingulum bundle. These changes are correlated with reduced reaction time. Gradient echo magnetic resonance imaging (MRI) may show microhemorrhages (Figure 16.2). Often, however, brain imaging is entirely normal.

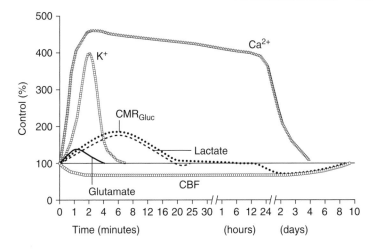

FIGURE 16.1 Neurometabolic cascade following concussion. CMR$_{Gluc}$ is the cerebral metabolic rate of glucose utilization. CBF is cerebral blood flow.

Source: Giza CC et al. In: Cantu RC, Cantu RI, eds. *Neurologic Athletic and Spine Injuries*. Philadelphia, PA:WB Saunders;2000:80–100.

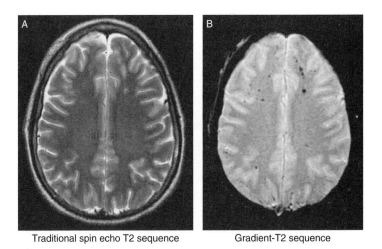

Traditional spin echo T2 sequence   Gradient-T2 sequence

FIGURE 16.2 Concussion and mild traumatic brain injury. Histology consistent with diffuse axonal injury has been noted in patients who died of other causes after mild concussion with no sequelae.

TABLE 16.2 Postconcussion Syndrome

Process 1—Early	Process 2—Late
■ Associated with MRI, PET, SPECT, and certain neuropsychological test abnormalities ■ Improvement may occur over several months ■ Deficits may persist even if studies are normal	■ Responsible for persistent headache, psychopathology, and some neurocognitive deficits ■ Often heralded by more severe early headache ■ May depend on pre-existing vulnerability ■ Possible mechanisms—windup, kindling, aberrant reinnervation ■ May be influenced by social and psychiatric factors

Abbreviations: MRI, magentic resonance imaging; PET, positron emission tomography; SPECT, single photon emission computed tomography.

To explain the fact that apparently very similar initial injury results in very different long-term outcomes, we believe that PCS is caused by two factors listed in Table 16.2.

Many tests may be done to evaluate PTH and posttraumatic syndrome. Unfortunately, the process of evaluation has been hijacked in our society by the medicolegal process and the need to blame. Brain imaging and

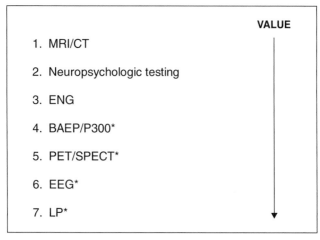

VALUE

1. MRI/CT

2. Neuropsychologic testing

3. ENG

4. BAEP/P300*

5. PET/SPECT*

6. EEG*

7. LP*

*of no value in routine testing.

FIGURE 16.3 Testing overview.

neuropsychological testing may be valuable in selecting therapy and determining progress. The use of other tests are fueled by the need to find "something" for medicolegal reasons or to lessen a patient's self-doubt but are not diagnostically useful and do not help in making treatment decisions (Figure 16.3).

Neuropsychological testing is often abnormal early but usually improves or resolves with time. The principal areas of abnormality are in the areas of information processing; auditory vigilance; reaction time; sustained, divided, and distributed attention; visual and verbal memory; design fluency; imagination; and analytic capacity.

The diagnosis of malingering is not made by exclusion because testing is normal or consistent with feigned illness. Patients may be observed performing tasks that they claim they are not able to perform. They may have worse performance than chance on forced choice memory test. Other characteristic findings include a personality disorder, such as an antisocial personality or borderline personality disorder, poor work history, prior claims for injury, or excessive endorsement of symptoms.

TREATMENT

What patients want first is an explanation of what is wrong, and second, they want symptom relief. They seek education including help in goal setting and achieving realistic expectations.

Nonpharmacologic interventions include psychological and emotional support; physical and manipulative therapies; occupational, speech, and vocational therapies; biofeedback and relaxation therapies; and cognitive-behavioral therapy. There are no successful controlled trials of medication treatment. Successful case series in PTH report intravenous dihydroergotamine and intravenous chlorpromazine as beneficial for short-term therapy. In uncontrolled studies, subcutaneous sumatriptan, amitriptyline, and occipital nerve blocks offer relief.

Success is best achieved by treating the headache with preventive and abortive medications like the primary headache it resembles, treating the comorbid and coexistent conditions, avoiding medication overuse, and encouraging nondrug therapies, for example, psychotherapy (especially short-term cognitive-behavioral therapy), biofeedback, physical therapy, massage, and Epley maneuver for positional vertigo. These therapies could be enhanced by pacing, relaxation skills, inviting family involvement, and providing education and support. Note that failure to respond to treatment is not evidence of psychogenicity.

REFERENCES

Cushing H. Subtemporal decompressive operations for the intracranial complications associated with bursting fractures of the skull. *Ann Surg.* 1908;47(5):641–644.

Evans RW, Rozen TD, Mechtler L. Neuroimaging and other diagnostic testing in headache. In: Silberstein SD, Lipton RB, Dodick DW, eds. *Wolff's Headache and Other Head Pain*. 8th ed. New York, NY: Oxford University Press;2008:63–93.

Vijayan N, Dreyfus PM. Posttraumatic dysautonomic cephalgia: clinical observations and treatment. *Trans Am Neurol Assoc*. 1974;99:260–262.

Young WB, Packard RC, Katsarava Z. Headaches associated with head trauma. In: Silberstein SD, Lipton RB, Dodick DW, eds. *Wolff's Headache and Other Head Pain*. 8th ed. New York, NY: Oxford University Press;2008:473–488.

17 Headache Associated with High and Low Cerebrospinal Fluid Pressure or Volume

INTRODUCTION

Disruption of the homeostasis of cerebrospinal fluid (CSF) often results in headache. Sometimes the features of the headache itself arouse clinical suspicion of this underlying cause, but often clinicians must rely on the history and the patient's characteristics to consider this in the differential diagnosis. Ultimately, diagnosis hinges on lumbar puncture to measure opening pressure. When it is normal, confirmatory tests to assess CSF volume and dynamics are required.

CSF PRODUCTION AND CIRCULATION

CSF is formed chiefly by choroid plexus in ventricles, and also may be formed transependymally in brain and spinal cord. Fluid circulates within and around the brain and spinal cord and is resorbed through the arachnoid villi into the major dural venous sinuses draining blood from the brain. About 500 mL per day is produced, with a total volume of 80 to 150 mL (Figure 17.1).

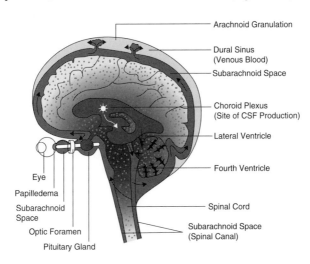

FIGURE 17.1 CSF circulation.
Source: http://www.ihrfoundation.org

INTRACRANIAL HYPERTENSION: PATHOGENESIS

Pressure is a function of volume (direct relationship) and compliance (inverse relationship). Elevated pressure can occur when too much fluid is produced or resorption through arachnoid villi is impaired. The latter can be a consequence of meningitis or subarachnoid hemorrhage. Reduced compliance (stiff brain/dura) is postulated to underlie idiopathic intracranial hypertension (IIH).

Why increased intracranial pressure causes headache is not clearly understood, but presumably it serves as an irritative stimulus to pain-sensitive intracranial structures, thus setting into motion the cascade of events underlying headache pathophysiology. As the diagram illustrates, papilledema arises because increased pressure is transmitted directly to the nerve head through the open optic nerve sheath.

INTRACRANIAL HYPERTENSION: CLINICAL FEATURES

Headache associated with elevated intracranial pressure and papilledema was previously called pseudotumor cerebri, so termed because the examiner is at first falsely led to believe that a brain neoplasm is the underlying cause. The "typical" patient is a young, obese female with a constant headache, often with migraine features, transient visual obscurations, and pulsatile tinnitus. However, in practice, cases of headache attributable to intracranial hypertension take on all forms and affect patients of both sexes, all ages, and all body types. The characteristics of the headache itself can range from featureless holocranial pressure to florid migrainous pain (unilateral, throbbing, associated with nausea, photophobia, and phonophobia). The headache may be worsened, alleviated, or unaffected by lying down. Intensity may vary predictably by time of day, may be constant, or may fluctuate randomly. There may be an antecedent history of episodic migraine or tension-type headache that evolved to a daily pattern, or a new type of headache may be superimposed on the old. Appropriate preventive medication trials usually fail, and subsequent medication overuse often occurs, which can also complicate the diagnosis. Papilledema need not be present, but venous pulsations may be absent. In such cases, the moniker "pseudotumor" is misleading, and it is, therefore, recommended to use terminology such as "intracranial hypertension." Sometimes a secondary cause can be identified, but in most cases, it is deemed IIH.

IDIOPATHIC INTRACRANIAL HYPERTENSION: DIFFERENTIAL DIAGNOSIS AND EVALUATION

When papilledema is present, ophthalmologic consultation and formal visual field testing are mandatory. When vision is threatened (enlarged blind spot precedes other gross visual field deficit precedes blindness), treatment is urgent.

Magnetic resonance imaging (MRI) may disclose pituitary flattening and stenosis of the venous sinuses, reflecting raised intracranial pressure. However, these findings are nonspecific. Slit-like ventricles have also been noted, but it is unclear whether this finding reflects reduced compliance of the CSF spaces or is an artifact of a recent lumbar puncture.

Lumbar puncture is diagnostic and can be therapeutic. Pressure must be measured with the patient in a relaxed lateral decubitus position. Normal pressure is 10 to 20 cm of CSF; 20 to 25 cm of CSF is a "gray zone," and more than 25 cm of CSF is considered high. Obese patients may have higher pressures at baseline (but this is controversial), so a higher threshold should be considered before final diagnosis. Similarly, thin patients tend to have lower pressures, so a reading of 20 to 25 cm CSF might be considered high in this scenario. CSF composition is usually normal and acellular, although low protein may be observed. Table 17.1 lists alternative diagnoses to be considered.

TABLE 17.1 IIH Differential Diagnosis

Brain tumor headache
Subdural hematoma
Hydrocephalus
Drug-induced intracranial hypertension (nonsteroidal anti-inflammatory drugs, minocycline)
Meningitic or postmeningitic intracranial hypertension (especially fungal)
Chronic migraine
Chronic tension-type headache
New daily persistent headache
Hemicrania continua
Medication overuse headache
Primary headache plus pseudopapilledema (congenitally anomalous discs)

Abbreviation: IIH, idiopathic intracranial hypertension.

INTRACRANIAL HYPERTENSION: TREATMENT

When elevated pressure is documented at lumbar puncture, enough fluid should be drained to attain a pressure of about 15 cm CSF. While fluid and pressure renormalize quickly, it is thought that lowering the pressure transiently can "reset" the circuit and relieve the headache.

Weight loss is the treatment of choice in overweight and obese individuals. Several medications have utility in treating IIH (Table 17.2), but the medication

TABLE 17.2 IIH Medications

Drug	Starting Dose	Target Dose	Side Effects	Monitoring/Comments
Acetazolamide	250 mg	2000–4000 mg/day, divided	Nausea, paresthesias	Watch for kidney stones
Furosemide	10 mg	40–80 mg	Hypotension	Monitor potassium
Hydrochlorothiazide	12.5 mg	25–50 mg	Hypotension	Antihypertensive effect diminishes over time
Spironolactone	25 mg	100–200 mg/day	Hypotension	Potassium sparing, monitor potassium, also used in PCOS
Topiramate	25 mg	600–1000 mg/day	Cognitive impairment, paresthesias, weight loss, hair loss, mood instability	Unproven effectiveness, weak carbonic anhydrase inhibitor, may also help by promoting weight loss, watch for kidney stones (calcium phosphate), narrow angle closure glaucoma

Abbreviations: IIH, idiopathic intracranial hypertension; PCOS, polycystic ovary syndrome.

of choice is the carbonic anhydrase inhibitor acetazolamide. Doses up to 3 or 4 g/day may be required. Topiramate also has carbonic anhydrase inhibiting activity, but very high doses (600–1000 mg/day) may be needed to achieve this effect. An added benefit of topiramate is the side effect of weight loss for obese patients. Many cannot tolerate the high doses of carbonic anhydrase inhibitors required to achieve lowering of CSF pressure, and adjunctive diuretics may be needed. Those used most commonly include furosemide, hydrochlorothiazide, and spironolactone.

When medical treatment is contraindicated or not tolerated, or when vision is imminently threatened and rapid intervention is required, procedural intervention may be necessary. Serial lumbar puncture can be an effective temporizing measure while awaiting the full effect of medication. Optic nerve sheath fenestration, in which tiny cuts are made in the dura around the optic nerve, can save vision in very urgent situations. The fenestrations provide an outlet for CSF under pressure, thus diverting it from the head of the optic nerve, and as healing occurs, the dura scars down and adheres to the nerve, thus eliminating the space in which fluid could accumulate and cause damage. While effective for saving vision, CSF pressure in the remainder of the system may not be affected, and therefore, headache does not always improve. Shunting (lumboperitoneal or ventriculoperitoneal) is another approach; however, there are often complications of infection, shunt failure, and overdrainage, making this a less desirable option.

CSF HYPOVOLEMIA: PATHOGENESIS

The inciting event is a leak within the CSF system, often of traumatic origin, such as occurs in lumbar puncture. Trauma to the head, neck, and back may also cause a leak, particularly in susceptible individuals (i.e., those with mixed connective tissue disorders, nerve sheath diverticula along the spine, or a thin cribriform plate). In some cases, the leak is spontaneous. Overdrainage from a shunting device is another cause.

One theory postulates that orthostatic head pain results from traction on the dura because of a lack of buoyancy: mechanical tension from gravitational forces activates meningeal nociceptors, which can then lead to the neuroinflammatory cascade that results in headache. There is no evidence to support this, however. Another theory proposes that the compensatory dilation of the thin-walled veins and venous sinuses, which are subjected to a transmural pressure gradient in the hypovolemic state, results in pain from stretch of these pain-sensitive structures. Another hypothesis pins the cause on increased compliance of the lumbar thecal sac. In the upright position, fluid falls into a floppy, highly compliant lumbar region (such as occurs with a tear in the dura and a low volume state), thus depleting rostral CSF spaces, resulting in the aforementioned reduced buoyancy and venous dilation.

TABLE 17.3 CSF Hypovolemia Headache Characteristics

■ Transformation over time	■ Second-half-of-the-day headache
■ Premonitory nonorthostatic headache	■ Worsened by exertion, cough, Valsalva
■ Thunderclap onset	■ Spontaneous remissions and recurrences
■ Paradoxically positional	

Abbreviation: CSF, cerebrospinal fluid.

CSF HYPOVOLEMIA: CLINICAL FEATURES

The hallmark of CSF hypovolemia is orthostatic headache, although it is not present in all cases. In fact, some patients have a nondescript headache, a reverse-orthostatic headache, or no headache at all. Nuchal and intrascapular pains are common accompaniments to head pain, and migrainous features may be prominent. Brainstem symptoms and signs may be present—a reflection of the sinking brain within an underpressured cranial vault. When extreme hypovolemia occurs, coma may ensue from hindbrain herniation. The onset of the syndrome is usually abrupt and may even be of thunderclap phenomenology. As in IIH, there may be an antecedent history of headache that resembles or evolves into the current headache, or the two may be completely different. Similarly, preventive trials may fail, and medication overuse often occurs (Tables 17.3 and 17.4).

TABLE 17.4 CSF Hypovolemia Nonheadache Characteristics

■ Nuchal or interscapular pain	■ Extrapyramidal or bulbar symptoms or signs
■ Nausea/vomiting (not necessarily orthostatic)	■ Galactorrhea, increased prolactin
■ Diplopia	■ Upper extremity radiculopathy
■ Hearing changes	■ Meniere-like syndrome
■ Photophobia, blurring, field cut	■ Incontinence
■ Facial numbness/weakness	■ Gait disturbance
■ Altered consciousness	

Abbreviation: CSF, cerebrospinal fluid.

CSF HYPOVOLEMIA: DIFFERENTIAL DIAGNOSIS AND EVALUATION

When the diagnosis is obvious based on history (e.g., orthostatic headache within a few days of lumbar puncture), it is probably best simply to treat empirically rather than confirm the diagnosis with further testing. Repeated lumbar puncture may only aggravate the condition, and neuroimaging is costly. Conservative management often results in complete resolution, but sometimes interventional treatment is required.

If the diagnosis is suspected based on history, the best noninvasive test to confirm it is MRI of the brain with gadolinium contrast. Findings consistent with CSF hypovolemia include sagging of the brain (which can be diagnosed erroneously as Arnold-Chiari malformation), pachymeningeal enhancement, engorgement of the pituitary gland, dilated venous sinuses, constriction of the superior ophthalmic vein, and subdural fluid collections. All of these changes are a physical reflection of decreased CSF pressure/volume within the cranium and illustrate the Monro-Kellie doctrine: lack of CSF is compensated by an increase in other space-occupying fluid. This most readily occurs via venous expansion, and is most notable in the large venous sinuses and the highly venous structures of the pachymeninges and pituitary gland. The superior ophthalmic vein, the conduit from extracranial venous drainage to intracranial venous drainage, becomes constricted because of increased flow velocities into the lower pressure space of the cranium (Bernoulli's principle). There is a limit to compensation, however, and eventually the brain sags noticeably, and when the condition is severe, subdural fluid accumulates. Similarly, in the spine, dural and venous changes may be seen on MRI, as well as potential sites of leak (i.e., nerve sheath diverticula), and occasionally, an actual leak may be seen (with heavily T2-weighted thin axial cuts) (Tables 17.5 to 17.7, Figures 17.2 to 17.4).

Not every case of CSF hypovolemia manifests with these findings on MRI. When CSF hypovolemia is suspected, but typical MRI findings are absent, lumbar puncture must be performed. Opening pressure should be measured in the lateral decubitus position. In some cases, pressure is so low that no reading can be obtained, and on rare occasions, pressure is negative (the practitioner will hear air being sucked through the needle into the CSF space). Opening pressure assessed in other positions (sitting or prone) is difficult to interpret (highly variable in the sitting position and potentially influenced by abdominal pressure in the prone position), and normal values are based on lateral decubitus measurements. However, it is useful to measure the opening pressure in both the lateral decubitus and sitting positions in order to calculate the

TABLE 17.5 CSF Hypovolemia Differential Diagnosis

Chronic migraine
Chronic tension-type headache
New daily persistent headache
Hemicrania continua
Medication overuse headache
Postural orthostatic tachycardia syndrome manifesting with headache
Carcinomatous meningitis

Abbreviation: CSF, cerebrospinal fluid.

TABLE 17.6 CSF Hypovolemia Brain MRI Findings

Pachymeningeal enhancement	Subdural fluid collections
Brain sag:	Engorgement of venous sinuses
False Chiari malformation	Pituitary enlargement
Effacement of cisterns	Small ventricles
Crowded posterior fossa	Elongation of brainstem
Flattened chiasm	Collapse of superior ophthalmic veins

Abbreviations: CSF, cerebrospinal fluid; MRI, magnetic resonance imaging.

TABLE 17.7 CSF Hypovolemia Spine MRI Findings

Extra-arachnoid fluid
Extradural extravasation of CSF
Nerve sheath diverticula
Pachymeningeal enhancement
Engorgement of venous plexus

Abbreviations: CSF, cerebrospinal fluid; MRI, magnetic resonance imaging.

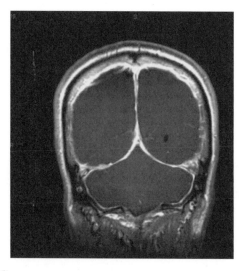

FIGURE 17.2 Pachymeningeal enhancement is best appreciated on coronal views, but usually can be seen easily in axial and sagittal views as well.

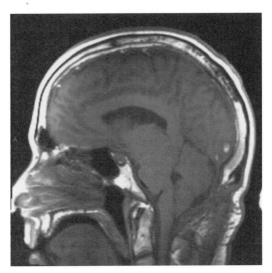

FIGURE 17.3 Note the cerebellar tonsillar herniation, flattening of the pons, and overall appearance of a wholly sunken brain. Also appreciated on the mid-sagittal T1 view (perhaps the most information-filled image in any brain MRI) is pituitary fullness. This patient errantly underwent suboccipital craniectomy for misdiagnosed Chiari-I malformation. The occipital lobe hyperintensities are remnants of embolic stroke due to patent foramen ovale (which, incidentally, was closed without improvement of the headache).

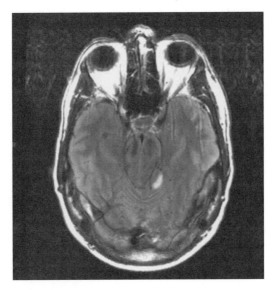

FIGURE 17.4 Most striking is the signal change in the choked, herniated bit of brain. Brainstem distortion is prominent, and sellar fullness is also appreciable.

hydrostatic indifferent point (HIP). The HIP is the point along the vertebral column where pressure is zero, and usually lies at the upper thoracic or lower cervical level in the upright position. By measuring the lumbar pressure in seated and decubitus positions, the HIP can be determined by the difference between the two pressures in centimeters of CSF. This number, in length in centimeters, is the distance above the needle in the sitting position where the HIP lies. In orthostatic headache, the HIP is lowered because of increased compliance in the lumbar region. (See Levine & Rapalino, 2001 for a detailed discussion). CSF composition is usually normal and acellular, although high protein may be observed.

Radionuclide cisternogram is the best confirmatory test when the diagnosis is suspected but uncertain (Figure 17.5). Lumbar puncture is performed as part of the procedure and allows for measurement of opening pressure. Radioactive tracer is injected into the CSF space and allowed to circulate. Images are obtained at 4 hours and 12 to 24 hours. The test demonstrates CSF dynamics. With normal CSF turnover, the tracer will begin to appear in the cranium at 4 hours and will reach the cerebral convexities by 12 to 24 hours, by which time the tracer will also have reached the kidneys and bladder. In CSF hypovolemia, turnover is rapid. At 4 hours, tracer already appears in the kidneys and bladder, and by 12 to 24 hours, it still has not reached the cerebral convexities, and may not even have risen above the foramen magnum. The

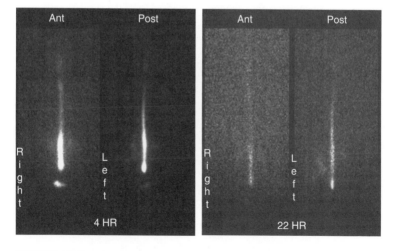

FIGURE 17.5 Nuclear cisternogram. Abnormal cisternogram demonstrates tracer in the kidneys/bladder after 4 hours, and failure of ascent of tracer to the cerebral convexities.

imaging resolution is low, so leaks along the spine often are not seen directly unless the leak is large. When nasal leaks are suspected, pledgets are inserted along the nasal turbinates and then removed at the end of the study. A high ratio of tracer on pledgets versus in blood indicates CSF leaking through the nose. In such cases wherein CSF rhinorrhea is suspected, every effort should be made to obtain a sample of the fluid from the nose, which can then be analyzed for the presence of β-transferrin, indicative of CSF.

The best test to localize a suspected leak is computed tomography (CT) myelogram/cisternogram. Like the radionuclide study, lumbar puncture is performed, and contrast is injected—in this case, radio-opaque iodinated contrast. Images are then obtained through the entire spine (and the skull when cranial leaks are suspected). This technique allows for direct visualization, in high resolution, of a leak, or a potential site of leak (such as nerve sheath diverticula). Images are obtained immediately and again after 3 to 4 hours if the leak is not detected. Very fast leaks are difficult to pinpoint as the contrast extravasates widely, but the fact that a leak is present will at least be proven. Very slow leaks are also difficult to locate because by the time enough fluid has extravasated to be detectible, the contrast medium has dissipated (it is gone after 4 hours) (Table 17.8).

MRI of the spine can be useful, but often fails to detect extravasation of spinal fluid unless the leak is substantial. Obtaining very heavily weighted T2 images in very thin axial cuts gives the best chance for detection. Still, this merely shows the distribution of CSF and does not demonstrate any dynamics. Very few centers perform magnetic resonance myelography/cisternography with gadolinium tracer. In principle, this is done the same way as CT myelography/cisternography. Advantages include lack or radiation exposure, safety in patients with allergy to iodinated contrast, and persistence of gadolinium within the CSF space for up to 72 hours to detect very slow leaks. Concerns have been raised regarding the safety of exposing the spinal cord directly to gadolinium, which could result in myelonecrosis.

Sometimes direct visualization at surgery is required. Again, lumbar puncture is performed, and fluouroscein is injected as the tracer. The suspected site of leak is exposed and inspected for fluouroscein. If seen, the defect is then corrected surgically.

TABLE 17.8 CSF Hypovolemia Types

Type I (Classic): +HA, abnormal MRI, low pressure
Type II (Normal Pressure): +HA, abnormal MRI, normal pressure
Type III (Normal Meninges): +HA, normal MRI, low pressure
Type IV (Acephalgic): −HA, abnormal MRI, low pressure

Abbreviations: CSF, cerebrospinal fluid; MRI, magnetic resonance imaging.

CSF HYPOVOLEMIA: TREATMENT

Conservative management involves flat bedrest, hydration, caffeine intake, and abdominal binders. Symptomatic headache medications are useful as a temporary measure until the syndrome is resolved. Sometimes intravenous administration of fluids, caffeine, and medication is required.

Failing this, blind lumbar epidural blood patch is usually successful, no matter where the site of leak lies. In this procedure, a needle is inserted into the epidural space, and 10 to 20 mL of the patient's own blood is injected. The name of the procedure is misleading, as the blood does not actually patch a hole, but rather, the fluid bolus serves to decrease compliance in the lumbar region, thus raising the HIP and relieving the orthostatic headache. This may also initiate inflammation to speed natural healing of the defect. In fact, any fluid could be used. Saline, dextran, and fibrin glue are common alternatives to blood. However, saline resorbs quickly, dextran is expensive, and fibrin glue, while it carries the added benefit of actually sealing a tear or rent, is a pooled blood product and carries the risk of transmissible disease (and also is costly). Sometimes a repeat patch is required, and sometimes it must be done at the level of leak. In refractory cases, it is reported that continuous epidural infusion of saline or dextran can resolve the condition, working in principle similar to the epidural patch.

For large defects, or bony defects, direct surgical repair may be required. Given enough time, even a large tear may heal completely, but surgical closure is definitive. For cases with increased lumbar compliance a novel surgical procedure involves removing a strip of dura along the length of the lumbar region then resealing the sac, thus reducing its compliance permanently. (Table 17.9)

In all cases, after treatment, vigilance should be maintained for the possible outcome of intracranial hypertension. In one unusual case, a man with a spontaneous leak from a ruptured diverticulum developed intracranial hypertension with papilledema after treatment. The high pressure eventually caused another

TABLE 17.9 CSF Hypovolemia Treatment Options

Bedrest	Epidural blood patch
(Over)hydration	Continuous epidural saline infusion
Caffeine	Epidural dextran
Theophylline	Epidural fibrin sealant
Abdominal binders	Intrathecal infusion
Steroids	Surgical repair
NSAIDs	

Abbreviations: CSF, cerebrospinal fluid; NSAIDs, nonsteroidal anti-inflammatory drugs.

leak to spring, and a delicate balance had to be achieved to maintain a normal pressure/volume state.

SUMMARY

Headaches attributable to derangements of CSF pressure/volume carry a wide range of clinical presentations. Sometimes one can mimic the other, or even become the other. Careful assessment and stepwise evaluation and treatment are the keys to success.

REFERENCES

Fishman RA. *Cerebrospinal Fluid in Diseases of the Nervous System*. Philadelphia, PA: W.B. Saunders Company; 1980.

Friedman DI. Idiopathic intracranial hypertension. *Curr Pain Headache Rep.* 2007;11(1):62–68.

Levine DN, Rapalino O. The pathophysiology of lumbar puncture headache. *J Neurol Sci.* 2001;192(1–2):1–8.

Mokri B. Spontaneous intracranial hypotension spontaneous CSF leaks. *Headache Currents.* 2005;2(1):11–22.

Schievink WI. A novel technique for treatment of intractable spontaneous intracranial hypotension: lumbar dural reduction surgery: brief communication. *Headache.* 2009;49(7):1047–1051.

18 Headaches and the Neck

Neck pain is a common feature in migraine. It can occur before, during, or after the head pain. Sixty-two percent of patients experience neck pain during the prodrome of migraine, 90% during the attack, and 41% during the postdrome. While patients may believe their migraine headaches are "caused" by their neck and should respond to cervical treatments, there is no evidence that such treatment is beneficial for long-term migraine management. Several criteria have been devised to help determine whether neck disease underlies a headache disorder.

ICHD-II CRITERIA

A. Pain, referred from a source in the neck and perceived in one or more regions of the head and/or face, fulfilling criteria C and D
B. Clinical, laboratory, and/or imaging evidence of a disorder or lesion within the cervical spine or soft tissues of the neck known to be, or generally accepted as, a valid cause of headache
C. Evidence that the pain can be attributed to the neck disorder or lesion based on one or more of the following:
   1. Demonstration of clinical signs that implicate a source of pain in the neck
   2. Abolition of headache following diagnostic blockade of a cervical structure or its nerve supply using placebo or other adequate controls
D. Pain resolves within 3 months after successful treatment of the causative disorder or lesion

Notably, the International Headache Society (IHS) specifically does not accept spondylosis as a cause of cervicogenic headache.

ANTONACCI CRITERIA

- Unilateral without side shift
- Symptoms of neck involvement—triggering, posture, shoulder or arm pain, reduced range of motion
- Moderate, nonexcruciating pain, episodic or continuous
- Pain starts in neck
- Anesthetic blockade abolishes pain, or close relationship to trauma
- May have autonomic symptoms, or migrainous symptoms

Several points in the Antonacci criteria deserve comment. A positive effect of anesthetic blockade from cervical muscle injection or occipital nerve block is common in migraine, so much so that a response to injection must be considered highly suggestive. Absence of a response to such injection with a positive response to a low-volume, anatomically precise injection aimed at a particular structure hypothesized to be causative (such as a facet injection) would be more helpful. Also, the allowance of autonomic or migrainous symptoms is problematic, as this implies involvement of structures that produce the symptoms of migraine or cluster headache.

SPECIFIC CAUSES OF CERVICOGENIC HEADACHE

Occipital Neuralgia

Occipital neuralgia is an overdiagnosed and uncommon disorder. The principal evidence for occipital neuralgia has always been a response to occipital nerve blocks. However, occipital nerve blocks are effective short-term treatments for migraine, which commonly manifest with occipital pain. In fact, many successful occipital nerve blocks actually anesthetize the nerve distal to the suspected site of pathology. Tenderness near or over the nerve could represent allodynia on the scalp or neck, or secondary muscle tenderness in the neck, which is nearly universal. The recent trend to perform exploratory surgery of the occipital nerve and subsequently diagnose nerve compression or other specific anatomical problems does not garner general acceptance, and a biological basis is unlikely. Short-term responses to this treatment are likely to represent the same neuromodulatory result that occipital nerve block or occipital nerve stimulation provides the migraine patient.

Nonetheless, true occipital neuralgia occasionally occurs, usually as a result of blunt, penetrating, or surgical trauma to the upper neck or occiput. The ICHD-II criteria, as outlined below, are worth noting:

A. Paroxysmal stabbing pain, with or without persistent aching between paroxysms, in the distribution(s) of the greater, lesser, and/or third occipital nerves
B. Tenderness over the affected nerve
C. Pain is eased temporarily by local anesthetic block of the nerve

In our opinion, tenderness is not particularly helpful, but a true Tinel's sign with tingling is.

Neck-Tongue Syndrome

This is a rare disorder with unilateral occipital pain and ipsilateral tongue numbness induced by rotation of the head. It is caused by subluxation of the atlanto-axial joint with stretching of the sensory branches of the C2 spinal nerve.

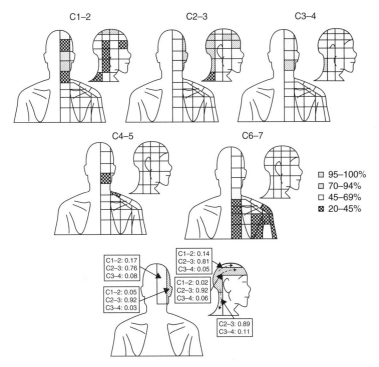

FIGURE 18.1 Areas of pain after irritation of zygapohyseal joint. The shading indicates the proportion of patients who perceived pain in the particular area indicated. *Source*: With permission from Cooper and colleagues, Blackwell Science.

Zygapophyseal Joint Pain (Facet Pain)

This is one of the more common causes of cervicogenic headache. Most people with facet pain have a history of trauma. Manual examination has been called into question as a diagnostic maneuver, although the facet joints can be theoretically stressed with hyperextension of a laterally bent neck. Each facet joint has a distinctive pain referral pattern (Figure 18.1).

Discogenic Pain is Controversial as a Source of Headache

A controversial source of pain in patients with headache is the intravertebral disc or the nerve root it compresses. Some studies have shown that stimulation of the C2–3 disc can cause a headache. However, the ICHD-II does not include this as a cause of headache, perhaps because it is rare. Herniated cervical discs below C2–3, which are much more common, generally should not be viewed as a cause of headache.

Myofascial Pain Syndrome

A trigger point is a hyperirritable spot within a taut band of a skeletal muscle. The spot is sensitive to pressure, which usually causes referred pain distant from the trigger point. Active trigger points cause local and referred pain and are responsible for at least part of the patient's symptoms. Trigger points in the temporalis, suboccipital, upper trapezius, and sternocleidomastoid muscles have been associated with episodic and tension-type headache. Each muscle has a distinctive referral pattern. Trigger point injections are used in patients with chronic neck pain and headache when the overall headache phenotype is chronic migraine. We inject 0.25 to 0.5 mL of 1% or 2% lidocaine or a mix of lidocaine with 0.5% bupivacaine, using a 30-gauge needle. We inject one third of the total volume, pull the needle partly out, and redirect it, and repeat, so as to create a triangle of injected local anesthetic within the trigger point. A muscle twitch may occur during the injection; this is characteristic of a trigger point.

REFERENCE

Simons DG, Travell J, Simons LS. *Travell and Simons' Myofascial Pain and Dysfunction: The Trigger Point Manual.* Vol 1. 2nd ed. Baltimore, MD: Williams & Wilkins; 1999.

19 Headache and the Nose and Sinuses: A Practical Approach

INTRODUCTION

Acute rhinosinusitis is a common medical condition that affects more than 30 million patients per year in the United States. The most common etiology is viral, but as many as 2% of cases result from, or develop into, bacterial infections. Bacterial sinusitis is overdiagnosed, but when it is present, it is commonly associated with headache and physical signs, such as purulent nasal discharge (Table 19.1). Pain, when present, is determined by the site of infection. Frontal headache and sinus pain, however, are common in patients with migraine or other primary headaches and respond to appropriate treatment.

TABLE 19.1 Common Signs and Symptoms in Acute Sinusitis

Purulent nasal discharge	Nasal congestion
Hyposmia or anosmia	Facial pain worse with bending forward
Fever or malaise	Maxillary tooth pain
Halitosis	Pain with mastication

PATHOPHYSIOLOGY AND ANATOMY

Nasal passages remove particulate matter and humidify inspired air. The paranasal sinuses communicate with the nasal airway and are lined by a ciliated epithelial layer and mucus. The ciliated epithelium clears mucus to the nasal airway, preventing bacterial contamination and infection. Obstruction of the sinus ostia (bony openings) can lead to an increase in carbon dioxide and an anaerobic environment that promotes bacterial growth. In chronic sinusitis, mucosal hyperplasia and nasal polyps sustain the disease.

Four major pairs of sinuses clear mucus or debris through their ostia. They are:

- *Maxillary sinuses*: The largest sinuses. Present at birth. Located behind the cheeks. Acute inflammation can cause pain in the cheeks, upper teeth, and jaw.

- *Ethmoid sinuses*: Located between the eyes, behind the bridge of the nose. Present and filled with fluid at birth but become pneumatized in the first year of life. Inflammation tends to cause pain behind the eyes and nose.
- *Frontal sinuses*: Located above the eyes. Develop at about 6 years of age. Inflammation may cause pain in the forehead.
- *Sphenoid sinus*: Located behind the eyes and nasal structures. Present at birth but pneumatization does not begin until around age 3. Inflammation may produce earache, deep aching at the vertex, and neck pain (Figure 19.1).

The cavernous sinuses, which are lateral to the sphenoid sinus on each side, contain the third, fourth, fifth, and sixth cranial nerves and the internal carotid arteries. Symptoms of cavernous sinus syndrome include ophthalmoplegia, proptosis, Horner syndrome, and trigeminal sensory loss. Potential causes include infection; inflammatory disorders, such as Tolosa-Hunt syndrome; vascular problems, such as internal carotid artery aneurysm; trauma; and neoplasm (Figure 19.2).

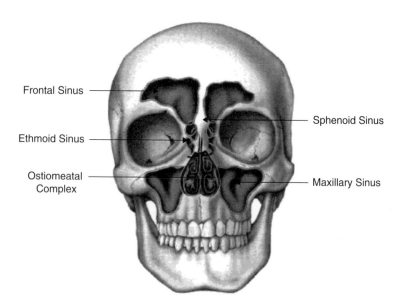

Frontal Sinus

Ethmoid Sinus

Ostiomeatal
Complex

Sphenoid Sinus

Maxillary Sinus

FIGURE 19.1 Sinus anatomy. The ostiomeatal complex, including the maxillary sinus ostium, infundibulum, middle turbinate, frontal ostium, and ethmoidal bulla, is a common drainage pathway for the frontal, maxillary, and ethmoid sinuses.

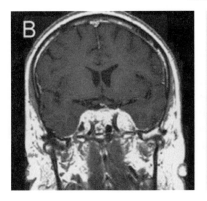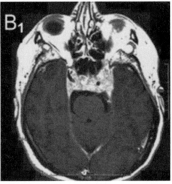

FIGURE 19.2 Cavernous sinus syndrome. Coronal and axial T2 weighted MRI showing bilateral cavernous sinus thickening due to actinomycosis. B is coronal, B₁ is axial
Source: From *Headache*. 2004; 44(8):803–11.

CLINICAL FEATURES

Rhinosinusitis is divided into four categories based on the time frame and symptoms of the disease. The categories are:

- *Acute rhinosinusitis*: 1 day to 4 weeks, usually viral if less than 7 days, often bacterial if more than 1 week, with complete resolution of symptoms
- *Recurrent rhinosinusitis*: Four or more episodes of at least 7 days in a year
- *Subacute rhinosinusitis*: 4 to 12 weeks
- *Chronic rhinosinusitis*: Signs or symptoms last longer than 12 weeks

Clinical symptoms and signs are helpful in making a diagnosis of sinusitis (Table 19.2), and the location of headache may predict the affected sinus. Headache location and severity, however, do *not* predict the presence of infection. Other symptoms, such as maxillary toothache, while more predictive of sinusitis, are less common. Acute sinusitis is a rare cause of thunderclap headache.

The most common causes of acute bacterial sinusitis are gram-positive cocci, such as *Streptococcus pneumoniae* or *Staphylococcus aureus*, and gram-negative organisms, such as *Moraxella catarrhalis*, *Haemophillis influenzae*, and *Escherichia coli*. Unlike most bacteria that cause acute sinusitis, *S aureus* is anaerobic and more common in chronic sinusitis. Nosocomial infections are common in patients after prolonged nasotracheal intubation and are usually caused by gram-negative bacteria, such as *Pseudomonas aeruginosa*, *Klebsiella pneumoniae*, *Enterobacter* species, or *Proteus mirabilis*. Most community-acquired sinusitis can be treated with narrow-

TABLE 19.2 Predictors of Rhinosinusitis

Major	Minor
Maxillary toothache	Cough
Abnormal transillumination	Ear pain/fullness
Purulent or colored nasal discharge	Halitosis
Poor response to decongestants	Headache
Fever (acute only)	Fatigue
Anosmia/hyposmia	Fever (chronic)
Facial pain/pressure [a]	

[a] Facial pain/pressure must be accompanied by other major nasal symptom or sign for the diagnosis of rhinosinusitis.

spectrum antibiotics, such as amoxicillin, and sometimes with topical glucocorticoids or decongestants. At times, broader spectrum antibiotics, such as amoxicillin-clavulanate, azithromycin, or fluroquinolones, may be needed. Besides treating the bacterial infection, treatment of sinusitis involves reducing swelling and promoting sinus drainage. Fungal rhinosinusitis is most common in diabetic or immunosuppressed patients and may require surgical debridement.

The most common risk factor for acute sinusitis is inflammation from a preceding viral infection, but systemic diseases, such as smoking or immune deficiency, place a patient at greater risk of serious infection (Table 19.3).

TABLE 19.3 Factors that Increase Risk of Sinusitis

Condition	Comments
Upper respiratory infection	Usually viral
Allergic rhinitis	Overuse of topical decongestants can make worse
Foreign bodies	Most common in children
Nasal polyps or tumors	
Cigarette smoking	
Deviated nasal septum	
Cystic fibrosis	Suspect *P aeruginosa*
Diabetes mellitus	Suspect fungal or *S aureus*
HIV infection	At higher risk for fungal, cytomegalovirus, mycobacterial, or parasitic infection

SPHENOID SINUSITIS

Maxillary, frontal, and ethmoid sinusitis are usually associated with nasal discharge and may be diagnosed with direct examination, endoscopy, or routine x-rays. Clinicians are usually able to identify most cases of sinusitis. However, about 3% of those with sinusitis have sphenoid sinusitis, which is often misdiagnosed because of its location. Symptoms such as postnasal drip or discharge are unusual. Usually sphenoid sinusitis occurs with pansinusitis, but it may occur alone, causing acute or subacute headache. Mucocele and neoplasm are potential noninfectious causes of sphenoid sinus disease. The clinical features of sphenoid sinusitis are variable and there are no specific pain features to alert clinicians to the diagnosis (Table 19.4). The treatment of sphenoid sinusitis may involve intravenous antibiotics.

Sinus infections, especially sphenoid sinusitis, may produce serious complications when the diagnosis is missed or treatment is ineffective. Complications include:

1. Orbital diseases (cellulitis, edema, abscess)
2. Epidural or cerebral abscess (Figure 19.3)
3. Meningitis
4. Superior sagittal sinus thrombosis
5. Cavernous sinus thrombosis, ophthalmoplegia
6. Pituitary insufficiency
7. Mucocele (retention cyst)

TABLE 19.4 Common Clinical Features of Sphenoid Sinusitis

Interferes with sleep	Progressive symptoms
Facial paresthesias	Fever
Visual loss/cranial nerve palsies	Not relieved with analgesics
Occipital, periorbital, or temporal (less often vertex) headache	Aggravated by standing, walking, bending, or coughing

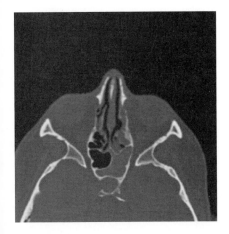

FIGURE 19.3 Sphenoid sinusitis. Sinus CT revealing inflammation of the left sphenoid and ethmoid sinuses.
Source: From *Headache*. 2007 Mar;47(3):463–6.

SINUSITIS: DIAGNOSTIC TESTING

Clinical features, such as sinus tenderness or colored, purulent nasal discharge, are helpful but not always diagnostic for sinusitis, especially sphenoid sinusitis. Routine rhinoscopy and sinus transillumination are often not sufficiently sensitive. Plain radiographs and sinus ultrasonography are of limited clinical value. Neuroimaging is indicated for diagnosis when chronic sinusitis is present or sphenoid sinusitis is suspected, and before endoscopy or surgery. Computed tomography (CT) and magnetic resonance imaging (MRI) are the most useful neuroimaging studies, although CT is generally the screening test of choice.

Advantages of CT in the evaluation of sinusitis include:

■ Defines the bony anatomy better than MRI
■ Gold standard for the diagnosis of sphenoid sinusitis
■ Coronal imaging effectively diagnoses ethmoid sinusitis
■ Adequately demonstrates mucosal thickening or air-fluid levels

Advantages of MRI in the evaluation of sinusitis include:

■ Better visualization of the nasal mucosa
■ Better than CT in distinguishing between bacterial, viral, or fungal infection
■ Distinguishes between mucoceles and benign tumors
■ Diagnoses bone erosion that is due to neoplasm

Nasal rhinoscopy allows direct visualization of nasal passages and sinus drainage areas and complements neuroimaging in the diagnosis of sinus disease. Advantages include:

■ Ability to detect disease missed on history, examination, or neuroimaging
■ Ability to obtain endoscopic cultures to identify organisms
■ Better assessment of patients with refractory or chronic symptoms

CONTACT POINT HEADACHE

Nasal septum deviation with a contact point on the lateral nasal wall (Figure 19.4) may occasionally produce episodic or transient headache. These abnormalities may be ignored by radiologists and should be considered in cases of headache refractory to standard therapy. ENT evaluation may be useful and intranasal blockade with an anesthetic, such as lidocaine, may confirm the diagnosis. If diagnosed correctly, removing the contact point may improve headaches. Since these radiologic abnormalities are common in patients without headache, it is unclear if contact point headache can occur without a central disorder, such as a genetic predisposition to migraine or headache.

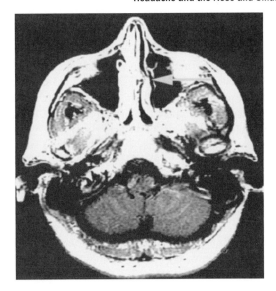

FIGURE 19.4 Contact point headache. Left nasal contact point in a patient with chronic migraine.
Source: From Rozen, *Neurology*, 2009:72;1107.

MIGRAINE AND "SINUS HEADACHE"

Although rhinosinusitis is common, significant headache is rarely a prominent feature and the sinuses themselves are relatively insensitive to pain. Because migraine, trigeminal autonomic cephalalgias, and other primary headaches often present with frontal, ocular, or facial pain, patients or clinicians may diagnose a "sinus headache" erroneously.

The International Classification of Headache Disorders, second edition (ICHD-II) defines headache attributed to rhinosinusitis as follows:

A. Frontal headache accompanied by pain in one or more regions of the face, ears, or teeth, fulfilling criteria C and D
B. Clinical, nasal endoscopic, CT and/or MRI imaging and/or laboratory evidence of acute or acute-on-chronic rhinosinusitis
C. Headache and facial pain develop simultaneously with onset or acute exacerbation of rhinosinusitis
D. Headache and/or facial pain resolve within 7 days after remission or successful treatment of acute or acute-on-chronic rhinosinusitis

The ICHD-II does not recognize chronic sinusitis as a cause of headache. Many patients or clinicians incorrectly diagnose primary headache disorders as "sinus headache" because of the location of the pain or parasympathetic symptoms that accompany attacks (Figure 19.5). Orbital or retro-orbital pain, rhinorrhea, nasal congestion, miosis, lacrimation, and facial sweating are common in both primary headache disorders and sinusitis. The proximity of parasympathetic nerves, which cause nasal symptoms, to the trigeminal nerves involved in migraine may explain this clinical overlap.

In fact, the vast majority of patients with self-described "sinus headache" have migraine (Figure 19.6). Most patients improve with various analgesics, including triptans. Cluster headache, other trigeminal autonomic cephalalgias, and hemicrania continua may also be misdiagnosed as sinusitis because of their frontal or orbital location and prominent autonomic features.

Although patients with chronic sinus symptoms often have primary headaches, clinicians must recognize bacterial sinusitis early to prevent complications (Table 19.5).

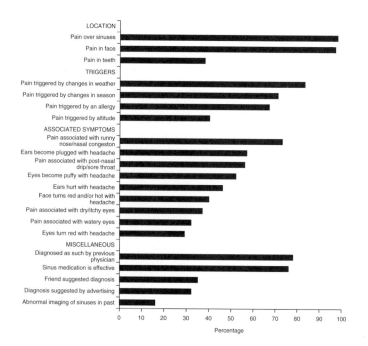

FIGURE 19.5 Symptoms of 100 patients with "sinus headache."
Source: From Eross et al., *Headache*. 2007.

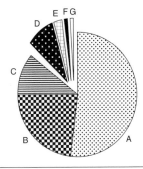

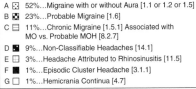

A ⊡ 52%…Migraine with or without Aura [1.1 or 1.2 or 1.5]
B ◪ 23%…Probable Migraine [1.6]
C ⊟ 11%…Chronic Migraine [1.5.1] Associated with MO vs. Probable MOH [8.2.7]
D ◪ 9%…Non-Classifiable Headaches [14.1]
E ☐ 3%…Headache Attributed to Rhinosinusitis [11.5]
F ■ 1%…Episodic Cluster Headache [3.1.1]
G ☐ 1%…Hemicrania Continua [4.7]

FIGURE 19.6 Actual ICHD-II diagnosis for 100 patients with "sinus headache."
Source: From Eross et al., *Headache*. 2007.

TABLE 19.5 Headache, Nasal, and Sinus Disease: Take-home Points

Sinusitis is usually associated with signs and symptoms, such as nasal discharge, other than headache

Acute rhinosinusitis < 1 week is usually viral

Sphenoid sinusitis is often missed based on history and physical examination and should be considered when patients have progressive or thunderclap headache and fever

Neuroimaging and endoscopy are complementary in the diagnosis of sinus disease

ICHD-II does not recognize chronic sinusitis as a cause of headache

Consider neuroimaging of the sinuses and ENT referral for patients with refractory or suspected "contact point" headache

"Sinus headache" is generally overdiagnosed by clinicians and patients

Most patients with chronic headache and sinus symptoms have a primary headache disorder such as migraine

REFERENCES

Cady RK, Dodick DW, Levine HL, et al. Sinus headache: a neurology, otolaryngology, allergy, and primary care consensus on diagnosis and treatment. *Mayo Clin Proc*. 2005;80(7):908–916.

Eross E, Dodick D, Eross M. The Sinus, Allergy and Migraine Study (SAMS). *Headache*. 2007;47(2):213–224.

Gupta M, Silberstein SD. Therapeutic options in the management of headache attributed to rhinosinusitis. *Expert Opin Pharmacother*. 2005;6(5):715–722.

Houser SM, Levine HL. Chronic daily headache: when to suspect sinus disease. *Curr Pain Headache Rep*. 2008;12(1):45–49.

Levine HL, Setzen M, Cady RK, et al. An otolaryngology, neurology, allergy, and primary care consensus on diagnosis and treatment of sinus headache. *Otolaryngol Head Neck Surg*. 2006;134(3):516–523.

Index